Marilyn,

All the best
to you!

Lisa Venn

Advocate's Guide to Improving Patient Experience

Third Edition

Published by Advocate Alliance
Cleveland, OH 44024 U.S.A

ISBN-13 978-1502303226

Author's Note

The regulatory references in this book are current as of this writing. However, regulations constantly change and patient advocates must ensure that they are relying upon up-to-date information. This book focuses on federal law. Patient advocates should seek advice from legal counsel to be certain of the laws, rules and requirements of their particular state or jurisdiction.

The purpose of this book is to highlight some of the most common issues encountered by patients and their advocates. This book is not intended as legal advice or comprehensive analysis of healthcare regulation. While the author has made every attempt to ensure that the information contained in this book is generally useful for its intended purposes, the author is not responsible for any error or omissions or for the results obtained through the use of this book.

Advocate's Guide to Improving Patient Experience

Third Edition

As always, I dedicate this book to advocates committed to improving patient experience

Contents

Contents (Cont.)

Advocate's Guide to Improving Patient Experience

Introduction

Recently I bought a car. Before setting foot on the dealership lot, I knew what cars were in stock, their sticker price, what the dealer paid for the cars, whether the cars had been in an accident, and whether the airbag deployed during that accident. I researched tricks of the car sales trade and armed myself with strategies to counter them. I knew the interest rates of car loans offered by the manufacturer and various banks. I researched my credit score and what interest rate I should expect. Having done my homework, I bought the car at the price and obtained a loan at the interest rate I desired.

To celebrate my fiftieth birthday, I made an appointment for a colonoscopy. I scheduled with a hospital close to home, with a physician who had privileges there, and made sure both providers were on my insurance plan. I drank the goop as directed in the "Prepping for your Colonoscopy" brochure and hoped for the best. Because the information was not available, I did not know whether that physician had done one or one hundred of these procedures, whether he did them well, what other patients thought about his care, or how much I would pay out-of-pocket for this unpleasant experience.

My experience shines a light on an unfortunate truth. Consumers have a better chance of buying the right car at the right price than selecting healthcare that best fits their needs. The lack of available information about the quality and cost of healthcare blindfolds patients attempting to choose wisely. Until very recently, we have been swinging in the dark.

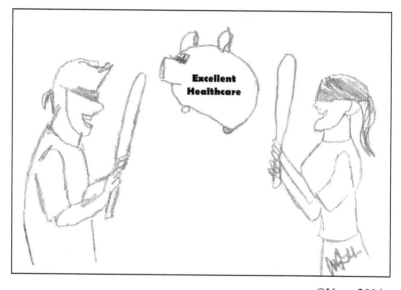

©Venn 2014

I have written this book to share good news: At long last, healthcare is changing into a consumer-friendly business, where resources are available to inform our choices. For the first time in the history of American healthcare, certain providers are required to measure and publicly report their quality outcomes and patient survey results.

We can now compare the quality scores of hospitals, nursing homes, and soon physicians, when choosing our providers. Likewise, before we select our insurance plan, we can review coverage details and quality ratings. Readily available resources allow us to select a substitute decision-maker and execute the documents to ensure our healthcare desires are followed. Recent laws strengthen patient rights, including the right to privacy and to receive a meaningful, timely response to complaints.

All of this wonderful information is only valuable if we know how to find it and what to do with it. Hence, this book is also a call to action. Improving our patient experience requires us to shift from passive recipients to informed healthcare consumers. It is not enough to simply be a patient. We must be empowered advocates: for ourselves and others, perhaps a child; an aging parent; an ailing life partner, friend, or neighbor.

Professionals such as lawyers, ombudsmen, social workers, case managers, physicians, and nurses, must vigorously advocate for their clients and patients.

This book provides advocates with tools necessary to obtain an excellent patient experience, which means the patient:

- ✓ makes informed decisions;
- ✓ participates in healthcare;
- ✓ understands patient rights; and
- ✓ resolves concerns.

Components of
Excellent Patient Experience

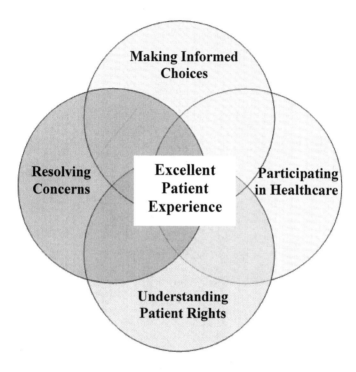

Part I
Making Informed Choices

Consumer choice based on reliable information about quality, customer satisfaction and price, is essential to keeping quality high and prices competitive. When customers have the ability to take their dollars elsewhere, businesses must provide high quality service at a competitive price or risk closure. The importance of choice based on quality, customer satisfaction, and cost is imbedded in the American psyche – except when it comes to healthcare.

Historically, healthcare providers such as hospitals, nursing homes, and physicians were immune to "free market" forces. Patients were not able to choose providers based on quality, price, and patient satisfaction because that information was not available. If patients were sick, they went to the doctor; if they were really sick, they went to the hospital. When choosing a hospital, patients could not ponder its rate of infection and quality outcomes because that information was neither measured nor publicly available. In the absence of quality data, government and private insurance plans paid providers regardless of the quality of care they provided. Even if a provider made a serious medical error resulting in patient harm, the government paid the bill. Thus, providers had no incentive to improve.

Not surprisingly the cost of healthcare skyrocketed, while the quality of care worsened. Healthcare was becoming like our old junker dripping oil in the driveway. We keep throwing money at it just to keep it running, hoping against hope it will pass its next e-check. At some point we need to stop our wasteful spending and come up with a new plan—either overhaul or scrap the resource-draining thing.

In healthcare, the new plan is called Value-based Purchasing.

Chapter 1
The Road to Value-based Purchasing

Since its beginning in 1965, Medicare (the federal health insurance program for people who are 65 or older, certain younger people with disabilities, and people with end-stage renal disease) paid healthcare providers whatever "reasonable" costs they charged to treat Medicare patients. This fee-for-service payment plan did not factor in the quality of or patients' opinions about the care they received. Instead it increased costs by rewarding providers for the volume and complexity of services they provided.[1]

This "You bill it, we pay it" reimbursement plan proved too expensive, devouring the Medicare coffers. The rising Medicare costs fueled by the aging population jeopardized the future of Medicare. To answer the threat, Medicare changed the way it paid for its beneficiaries' hospital care. In 1983, Medicare switched from fee-for-service to a prospective payment system (PPS), which means that it pays hospitals a pre-determined, set rate based on the patient's diagnosis. If the cost of the patient's treatment is less than the set rate, the provider profits; if the cost is greater, the provider loses money.

Medicare also changed the way it paid nursing homes and home health services. In 1997, after a period of rapid growth in Medicare nursing home expenditures, Medicare implemented a PPS to reimburse sub-acute services given in nursing homes.

Effective October 1, 2000, Medicare pays home health agencies a predetermined base rate, adjusted for the health condition and care needs of the Medicare beneficiary.

While changing the payment scheme saved money in the short-term, it did not improve the quality of care.

In its 1999 landmark report *To Err is Human: Building a Safer Health System*[2] the Quality of Care in America Committee of the Institute of Medicine (IOM) reported that as many as 98,000 people die in hospitals each year as a result of preventable medical errors. The IOM called for a nationwide mandatory reporting system by which certain healthcare providers would voluntarily report adverse events. The IOM also recommended that purchasers of healthcare (both private and government) consider the quality of providers when buying services.

Purchasing healthcare based on quality of providers was not possible at the time of the IOM report because there was no reliable data upon which to make a decision.

The government realized that in order to improve the quality of healthcare, three things must happen. First, healthcare providers must measure and report quality outcomes and patient satisfaction scores. Second, these scores must be publicly available so consumers and payors can make informed choices; and finally, providers' payment must be tied to quality and patient satisfaction scores.

The Patient Protection and Affordable Care Act of 2010 (Affordable Care Act)[3] established the Hospital Value-based Purchasing (VBP) Program. Starting October 1, 2012, hospitals are rewarded for how well they perform on a set of quality measures as well as on how much they improve in performance relative to a baseline. Quality measures fall into five clinical areas: heart attack; heart failure; pneumonia; surgical care; and healthcare associated infections.[4]   VBP also factors in the mortality (the rate of death) within 30-days of discharge for heart attack, heart failure, or pneumonia.   Providers with the highest or most improved quality scores will receive higher Medicare reimbursement.

The Affordable Care Act also requires the Center for Medicare & Medicaid Services (CMS) to develop Value-based Purchasing programs for home health agencies, skilled nursing facilities, ambulatory surgical centers, specialty hospitals (such as long-term care facilities), and hospice programs. Beginning in 2015, CMS will pay certain physicians based on the quality of their services. By 2017 Physician Value-based Purchasing (PVBP) will apply to all physicians.

In addition to requiring Medicare certified hospitals to report these quality and clinical outcomes, CMS mandates that hospitals survey every adult patient discharged from the hospital.[5]

The survey, called the Hospital Consumer Assessment of Healthcare Providers and Systems (HCAHPS),[6] asks patients to rate their experience in eight categories:

- ✓ Nurse communication;
- ✓ Doctor communication;
- ✓ Responsiveness of hospital staff;
- ✓ Pain management;
- ✓ Communication about medications;
- ✓ Cleanliness and quietness of hospital environment;
- ✓ Discharge information; and
- ✓ Overall rating of hospital

The Affordable Care Act mandates that CMS require other healthcare providers to survey patients about their experience with that provider. Presently, certain clinician and physician groups are voluntarily surveying their patients.[7] By 2015, CMS will mandate that all physician groups and individuals survey their patients. CMS will publicly report those results.

Some private insurers are following the federal government's lead, determining reimbursement rates based on evidence of quality care.

Value-based Purchasing: Refusing to Pay for Avoidable Errors

In 2002, the National Quality Forum (NQF) published a report, *Serious Reportable Events in Healthcare,*[8] which identified 27 adverse events that are serious, largely preventable, and of concern to both the public and healthcare providers.

At the time of the NQF report and six years beyond, Medicare reimbursed hospitals in full for their mistakes. For instance, if during a Medicare beneficiary's hospital admission for hip surgery, he developed a very bad bedsore, contracted an infection, and fell, breaking his other hip, Medicare paid the entire bill. This arguably perverse incentive came to an end in 2008 when CMS stopped paying for certain preventable Hospital Acquired Conditions (HACs). As of 2013, HACs include:

> ➢ Foreign Object Retained After Surgery
> ➢ Air Embolism
> ➢ Blood Incompatibility
> ➢ Stage III and IV Pressure Ulcers
> ➢ Falls and Trauma
> ➢ Manifestations of Poor Glycemic Control
> ➢ Catheter-Associated Urinary Tract Infection (UTI)
> ➢ Vascular Catheter-Associated Infection
> ➢ Surgical Site Infection, Mediastinitis, Following Coronary Artery Bypass Graft (CABG):
> ➢ Surgical Site Infection Following Bariatric Surgery for Obesity
> ➢ Surgical Site Infection Following Certain Orthopedic Procedures
> ➢ Deep Vein Thrombosis (DVT)/Pulmonary Embolism (PE) Following Certain Orthopedic Procedures[9]

Many private insurance companies have followed the government's lead and no longer pay for medical errors.

Improving Patient Care through Value-based Purchasing: The Story of Hospital Readmissions

Hospital readmission rates demonstrate how payment influences quality. During the heyday of fee-for-service reimbursement, Medicare paid for a patient's hospital stay with few limitations. As the population aged, more Medicare patients were hospitalized and Medicare costs soared. To stem healthcare costs, Medicare changed how it pays for hospital care from fee-for-service to a Diagnostic-Related Group (DRG) system, providing hospitals a lump sum to provide care to each patient. Hospitals profit if the cost of care is less than the DRG payment, thus incentivizing hospitals to discharge the patient sooner rather than later. Many of these patients, discharged before medically ready, returned to the hospital within 30 days of discharge.

The cost of caring for patients readmitted to the hospital soon after discharge strained the Medicare budget. In its 2007 report, the Medicare Payment Advisory Commission (MedPAC) reported that 17.6% of hospital admissions resulted in readmissions within 30 days of discharge at a cost of $15 billion.[10]

To roll-back the readmission rate and reduce Medicare costs, CMS required hospitals to track and report their readmission rates. Beginning 2008, CMS began reporting hospitals' readmission rates on Medicare's Hospital Compare website.[11] As of 2012, CMS financially penalizes hospitals that have high readmission rates for patients with conditions of heart attack, heart failure, and pneumonia.

For fiscal year 2014, CMS added (1) patients admitted for an acute exacerbation of chronic obstructive pulmonary disease (COPD); and (2) patients admitted for elective total hip arthroplasty (THA) and total knee arthroplasty (TKA).[12]

In its June 2013 Report to Congress, MedPac advised that since the implementation of Value-based Purchasing, the Medicare beneficiary readmission rate has declined.[13]

MedPac encouraged Congress to continue the readmission reduction program, suggesting further refinements to improve incentives for hospitals and generate program savings through reduced readmissions rather than higher penalties.

Chapter 2
Choosing Our Healthcare Providers

The first step to experiencing excellent care is to choose our healthcare providers and health insurance plan based on solid information. Making these choices can feel overwhelming because healthcare is complex, highly regulated and expensive. Even those of us committed to making sense of it all can be baffled by the overabundance of information. For instance, an Internet search "How to choose a healthcare provider" yielded 11,200,000 results; "How to choose a health plan" produced 178,000,000 hits.

Despite the challenge, empowered advocates must strive to make informed choices *before* a healthcare crisis happens. When chest pain strikes at 2:00 a.m., requiring an immediate trip to the emergency department, there is no time to Google one's options. Instead, we must seize the opportunity to make advance healthcare decisions based on available information. When we choose providers based on the quality of care they provide, patients' opinions about them, and cost, we increase the likelihood that we will be satisfied with our decision. Similarly, we are empowered consumers when we choose our insurance plan understanding what the plan covers and what we will pay out-of-pocket for our care. Our informed choices have the potential of improving our experience and improving healthcare as a whole.

When we reward the good providers with our business, steering clear of the poor performers, we have the ability to affect the market.

Choosing Providers Based on Quality Measures, Outcomes and Patient Experience Scores

CMS Hospital Compare website allows consumers to compare the quality and patient experience scores of several hospitals to help make an informed choice. Information available at www.hospitalcompare.hhs.gov includes:

- Timely and effective care:
  - ➢ How often and quickly each hospital gives recommended treatments for certain conditions like heart attack, heart failure, pneumonia, children's asthma, stroke and blood clots, and follows best practices to prevent surgical complications.
- Readmissions, complications, and deaths:
  - ➢ How each hospital's performance on the readmission and morality (death) measures compares to the national rate.
  - ➢ How likely patients will suffer from complications while in the hospital or after undergoing certain inpatient surgical procedures.
  - ➢ How often patients in the hospital get certain serious conditions that could have been prevented if the hospital followed procedures based on best practices and scientific evidence.
- Use of medical imaging:
  - ➢ How a hospital uses outpatient services such as CT scans and MRIs.

- Patients' survey scores
- Number of Medicare patients:
  - How many people with Medicare have had certain procedures or have been treated for certain conditions at each hospital.
- Medicare payment:
  - Information about how much Medicare pays hospitals.[14]

The public availability of this patient experience data is changing the way hospitals deliver service.

I recently visited a friend admitted to a community hospital, which was notorious for poor service. I was delighted to see its newfound efforts to provide excellent patient experience. A nurse frequently checked to ensure the call light was in reach and the patient knew how to use it. Nurses and doctors explained the purpose of medications and the risks and benefits of tests and procedures. The television listed a menu item: "My room is too noisy to sleep." By clicking this option, the patient signals the nursing station of the issue. The nurse offers to provide a white noise machine, ear plugs, and/or to close the patient's door. Additionally, the patient's "It's too noisy" menu selection is electronically recorded and provided to the hospital administration for review and quality improvement.

The hospital's new consumer-friendly approach is likely related to the fact that patients' opinions about their hospital experience affect hospital payment.

CMS Physician Compare website allows consumers to find individual physicians or groups based on location and specialties. CMS intends to post performance rating information beginning in 2015. The information is available at:

http://www.medicare.gov/physiciancompare

CMS Nursing Home Compare website allows consumers to compare data about nursing home characteristics, health deficiencies issued during the three most recent state inspections, complaint investigations, staffing data and penalties levied against nursing homes. Quality measures data is reported by the nursing homes and neither the state nor federal surveyors review it for accuracy, hence CMS warns consumers to interpret the data cautiously. The information is available at:

http://www.medicare.gov/nursinghomecompare

CMS Home Health Compare website allows consumers to compare quality and patient experience data about home healthcare providers. All Medicare certified home health agencies serving 60 or more patients are required to report certain quality data.

The available home health data includes:

- *Process measures* such as how often the home health team:
  - ➢ began their patients' care in a timely manner;
  - ➢ determined whether patients received a flu shot for the current flu season; and
  - ➢ for patients with diabetes, got doctor's orders, gave foot care, and taught patients about foot care.

- *Outcome measures* such as how often patients:
  - ➢ got better at walking or moving around.
  - ➢ got better at getting in and out of bed.
  - ➢ had less pain when moving around.
  - ➢ experienced improved or healed wound care after an operation.[15]

- *Patient responses* to questions including:
  - ➢ How often did the home health team give care in a professional way?
  - ➢ How well did the home health team communicate with patients?
  - ➢ Did the home health team discuss medicines, pain, and home safety with patients?
  - ➢ Would patients recommend the home health agency to friends and family?
  - ➢ How would patients rate the overall care from the home health agency?

The information is available at:

http://www.medicare.gov/homehealthcompare

CMS Dialysis Facility Compare website allows consumers to compare quality data about dialysis facilities. Measures reported on the website include information about:

- anemia management;
- dialysis adequacy;
- vascular access;
- mineral and bone disorder;
- rate of hospital admission; and
- patient death rate[16]

The information is available at:
http://www.medicare.gov/dialysisfacilitycompare

In an effort to help consumers make informed decisions and improve the quality of healthcare, CMS requires certain providers to measure and report quality measures, outcomes, and patient survey results. If consumers use the available information to make healthcare choices, providers will recognize that data affects their bottom line. They will improve the quality of the care and service they provide, or risk closure.

Choosing Providers Based on Cost

Imagine shopping for a washer and dryer and being told by the salesperson that he is not able to tell you the cost, but will send you the bill after you make your purchase. Not one of us would buy the appliances or return to that store. Yet in healthcare, this scenario plays out every day as it is all but impossible to obtain an accurate statement of what a particular healthcare service will cost us. We first learn what we owe when we receive the bill.

When asked by a patient how much a particular service will cost, healthcare providers typically advise it is not possible to calculate the cost because there is no way to predict what services the patient will need or to know the specifics of the patient's insurance coverage. Providers will direct the patient to speak with the insurance plan representative who will advise there is no way to calculate the cost without knowing exactly what services will be performed and whether the providers are in or out of network.[17]

The lack of price transparency is particularly troubling as individuals shoulder a larger share of the healthcare costs by way of deductibles and copayments. According to the Kaiser Family Foundation, the 2013 annual premium for employer-sponsored family health coverage reached $16,351, an increase of 4 percent from 2012. Workers on average pay $4,565 towards the cost of their coverage. Over the last 10 years, the average premium for family coverage has increased 80%.[18]

In its 2011 report, the Government Accountability Office (GAO) concluded that consumers can make the most meaningful choices only when they know their "complete health care cost," defined as price information on a healthcare service or services that:

- ✓ reflects discounts negotiated between the provider and the payor;
- ✓ includes all costs to the consumer associated with a service or services, including hospital, physician, and lab fees; and
- ✓ identifies a consumer's out-of-pocket costs.[19]

As a nation, we are inching toward price transparency. The Affordable Care Act requires hospitals operating in the United States to annually make public and update a list of their hospital's standard charges for items and services they provide.[20]

Recently CMS posted payment data for common procedures performed in hospitals, ambulatory surgery centers, and physician offices.[21] Additionally, CMS' online Medicare Part D Plan Finder provides information on prescription drug prices. A Medicare beneficiary enters the name and dosage of a drug and the database provides the expected out-of-pocket costs.

30 states have laws requiring some level of price disclosure, yet most of those laws are woefully inadequate to protect consumers.

In its March 25, 2014 *Report Card on State Price Transparency Laws,*[22] the Catalyst for Payment Reform graded all 50 states on their levels of price transparency.

To earn an "A," (the highest score), a state must mandate posting of a broad range of:

✓ providers (facility and practitioner);

✓ prices (paid and charge amounts); and

✓ scope of services (all inpatient and outpatient).

No state received an A; two states (Maine and Massachusetts) received a B; three states received a C; and 45 states received an F.

These results are unacceptable. We expect to see the exact price of our morning Cafè Mocha listed on the marquee of our favorite coffee shop.   We must demand that our state and federal government require healthcare to demonstrate similar cost transparency.

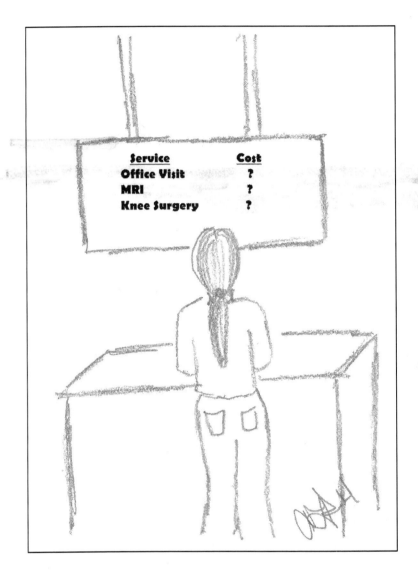

Choosing Providers Based on their Lack of Conflicts of Interest

When a healthcare provider such as a physician or hospital has a financial relationship with an outside company such as a pharmaceutical or a medical device manufacturer, that relationship may threaten the provider's objectivity when making decisions for the patient. For instance, studies have shown that physicians who receive something of value from a pharmaceutical company are more likely to prescribe that company's drug.[23]

In response, Congress passed the Physician Payments Sunshine Act (PPSA). Beginning August 2014, pharmaceutical companies and medical device companies must publically report money and other things of value given to teaching hospitals and physicians.

CMS will post these payments on a public website.[24]

To address potential conflicts of interest, CMS also requires certain healthcare providers to disclose a conflict of interest to the patient.

Physician-owned hospitals are required to disclose to their patients the names of the physician owners and the names of immediate family members of the physician who have an ownership or investment interest in the hospital. Additionally, physicians are required to disclose to their patients at the time of referral if they (or their immediate family members) have an ownership or investment interest in the hospitals to which they refer patients for treatment.[25]

When preparing for a patient's discharge, a hospital must inform the patient or the patient's family of their freedom to choose among participating Medicare post-acute providers (home health agencies and skilled nursing facilities). The hospital must disclose any financial interest in the post-acute facility.[26]

Knowing whether the provider has a real or potential conflict of interest is just one piece of the puzzle. When we also have access to quality data, patient survey results, and information about cost, we are in the best position to choose healthcare that meets our needs.

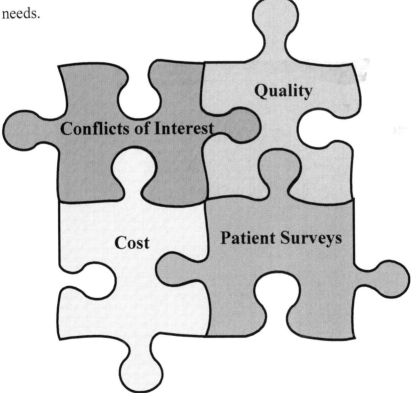

Chapter 3

Choosing Our Health Insurance Plan

The health plan we choose will affect our healthcare options and the amount we pay out-of-pocket. Insurance coverage types include employment-based; direct-purchase; and government, such as Medicare, Medicaid (state and federally funded health insurance for low income persons), and military. When choosing a plan, we must determine:

1. What the plan covers;
2. What the plan costs;
3. Which healthcare providers are on the plan; and
4. How the insurance plan is ranked.[27]

1. What the Plan Covers

Under the Affordable Care Act all health plans sold to *individuals* and *small businesses* must cover:

- ✓ ambulatory patient services;
- ✓ emergency services;
- ✓ hospitalization;
- ✓ maternity and newborn care;
- ✓ mental health and substance use disorder services, including behavioral health treatment;
- ✓ prescription drugs;
- ✓ rehabilitative and habilitative[28] services and devices;
- ✓ laboratory services;
- ✓ preventive and wellness services and chronic disease management; and
- ✓ pediatric services, including oral and vision care.[29]

The Affordable Care Act adds many protections related to *employment-based group health plans*, such as:

- ✓ Extending dependent coverage up to age 26;
- ✓ Prohibiting preexisting condition exclusions for children under age 19 and for all individuals beginning in 2014;
- ✓ Requiring easy-to-understand summaries of a health plan's benefits and coverage;
- ✓ Prohibiting annual or lifetime payout caps;
- ✓ Requiring coverage for certain preventive services (such as blood pressure, diabetes and cholesterol tests, regular well-baby and well-child visits, routine vaccinations and many cancer screenings) without cost-sharing; and
- ✓ Mandating coverage of emergency services in an emergency department of a hospital outside the health plan's network without prior approval from the health plan.

To learn more about these rights visit the Department of Labor website: http://www.dol.gov/ebsa/healthreform/consumer.html

2. What the Plan Costs

Out-of-pocket costs include the monthly premium we pay for the insurance, deductibles, and copayments. The deductible is the amount we pay for healthcare or prescriptions before our insurance or prescription drug plan begins to pay. The copayments are the amount we pay for each service. Generally, if we choose a plan with a higher premium, we will pay less out-of-pocket for medical care.

If we receive insurance through our employer, cost information will be on the Summary of Care Benefits form.

Medicare beneficiaries can obtain information regarding coverage and cost by reading the *Medicare & You 2014* publication. Medicare provides this booklet annually and it is available online at Medicare.gov.

If we buy insurance through our state marketplace, we will be able to see and compare the cost-sharing structure of plans before we buy. The four Affordable Care Act "metal plans" (bronze, silver, gold, and platinum) are defined by the percentage of medical expenses they cover. Bronze plans cover 60% of covered medical expenses for a typical enrollee population, silver plans 70%, gold plans 80%, and platinum plans 90%. We can find the average out-of-pocket costs for medical services for each metal plan category online at Healthcare.gov.[30]

3. Which Healthcare Providers are on the Plan

Every health insurance plan has a network of providers, such as doctors, hospitals, laboratories, imaging centers, and pharmacies, that have signed contracts with the insurance company agreeing to provide their services to plan members at a specific price.

If our healthcare provider is not in our health plan network, we may have to pay all or a significant part of the bill. If we have certain providers we want to continue to use, we must make sure they are in the health plan network. It is up to us, not our provider, to know who is and is not in our health plan network. We must keep in mind that the providers participating in our insurance plan may change throughout the years.

If we have employer-based insurance, we can obtain a provider list from the health plan or our employer. If we are considering a metal plan through our state Health Insurance Marketplace, there may be links to the provider directory on its website.

4. How the Insurance Plan is Ranked

The National Committee for Quality Assurance (NCQA) ranks health plans based on clinical performance, member satisfaction and results from NCQA accreditation surveys. Plan participation in the ranking is voluntary. Hence, if we do not see our plan it may be that the plan did not submit data, or did not have enough data to be ranked, or did not agree to have the data disclosed to the public.

The NCQA insurance plan rankings are available at:
http://www.ncqa.org/ReportCards/HealthPlans/HealthInsurancePla
nRankings.aspx

Chapter 4

Selecting a Substitute Decision-Maker

Every patient needs an advocate who can help obtain high quality, affordable healthcare, and resolve concerns. Ideally we are our own best advocate. It is wise, however, to select a substitute decision-maker in the event that we become unable to make informed medical decisions for ourselves. While not required to do so, each of us should indicate--in written form--our healthcare desires, and identify a decision-maker in the event we are not able to speak for ourselves.

Self-determination and the Right to Make Informed Decisions

The right to give or withhold informed consent is rooted in common law principles, state and federal laws, and clinician Codes of Ethics. Patients' right to make informed decisions includes the right to:

- ✓ receive sufficient information to enable them to weigh the risks and benefits of consenting to or refusing certain treatments and procedures;
- ✓ be informed of their health status; and
- ✓ be involved in care planning and treatment.

CMS requires healthcare providers to inform patients or their legal representative of anticipated benefits, material risks, and alternative therapies; to inform patients of their health status; and involve patients in their care planning and treatment.[31]

The Patient Self-Determination Act

Self-determination is the basic principle upon which all healthcare decision-making rests. The law recognizes a person's right to control decisions affecting his or her care and treatment.

On November 5, 1990, Congress passed the Patient Self-Determination Act (PSDA).[32] The PSDA requires Medicare and Medicaid providers (hospitals, critical access hospitals, skilled nursing facilities, nursing facilities, home health agencies, providers of home healthcare and Medicaid personal care services, hospices, and religious nonmedical healthcare institutions) to maintain written policies and procedures concerning advance directives with respect to all adult individuals receiving medical care. These providers must provide the individuals with information regarding:

- ✓ the right to participate in and direct their own healthcare decisions;
- ✓ the right to accept or refuse medical or surgical treatment;
- ✓ the right to prepare an advance directive (discussed on the following pages); and
- ✓ the provider's policies that govern the utilization of these rights.

The PSDA also prohibits institutions from discriminating against a patient who does not have an advance directive. The PSDA requires institutions to document in the patient record whether or not the patient has executed an advance directive. Institutions must provide ongoing community education on advance directives.

Advance Directive

An advance directive is a written instruction such as a living will or durable power of attorney for healthcare, recognized under state law, relating to the provision of healthcare when the individual is incapacitated.

State law governs the procedural requirements pertaining to advance directives. Most states give an individual the right to execute advance directives to take effect if and when he or she becomes unable to make his or her own medical decisions. Types of advance directives include a durable power of attorney for healthcare, a living will, a Do Not Resuscitate (DNR) order, and an anatomical gift.

Durable Power of Attorney for Healthcare

A durable power of attorney for healthcare allows an individual (called the principal) to name someone (called the agent or attorney in fact) to make medical decisions when the principal is no longer capable. The agent's authority springs into effect only when the principal's physician determines that the principal does not have the capacity to make his or her own medical decisions.

Living Will

A living will is a document that details one's wishes regarding the degree and amount of healthcare desired should one become mentally incapable of making or communicating healthcare decisions.

Do Not Resuscitate (DNR) Order

A DNR order is an advance directive that is to be followed when a person's heart or breathing stops and he or she is unable to communicate his or her wishes regarding treatment. Laws pertaining to DNR orders vary by state.

The National Hospice and Palliative Care Organization (NHPCO), an excellent resource for end of life decision-making, is available online at: http://www.nhpco.org.

Anatomical Gift

An anatomical gift is a donation of all or part of a human body to take effect after the donor's death for the purpose of transplantation, therapy, research, or education.

Advocate's Checklist:

Before a healthcare crisis:

✓ *Choose healthcare providers*
✓ *Choose health insurance*
✓ *Select a substitute decision-maker*

Part II

Actively Participating in Our Healthcare

In Part I of this book, we discussed improving the patient experience by shifting from passive recipients to informed healthcare consumers. We discussed how to choose our healthcare providers, insurance plan, and substitute healthcare decision-maker. In Part II, we discuss how to improve the patient experience by actively participating in our healthcare and:

- ✓ staying healthy;
- ✓ using reliable sources to manage our health; and
- ✓ preparing for our appointments.

Ideally, we maintain a healthy lifestyle so that our need for the healthcare system is preventative. Should we face a medical diagnosis requiring medical management, however, we owe it to ourselves to become fully knowledgeable about our condition. This will better prepare us to navigate the road to recovery.

Chapter 1
Staying Healthy

It is comforting to know that there is much we can do and plenty of information to help us stay healthy. While there are no guarantees that a healthy lifestyle will shield us from all health problems, science has identified lifestyle changes we can make to significantly lessen our health risks.

As reported in *Pharmaceutical Research*,[33] 90–95% of cancer cases have their roots in the environment and lifestyle. The lifestyle factors include: cigarette smoking, diet (fried foods, red meat), alcohol, sun exposure, environmental pollutants, infections, stress, obesity, and physical inactivity.

The researchers conclude that to prevent cancer we must:

- ✓ quit smoking;
- ✓ eat more fruits and vegetables;
- ✓ eat minimal meat;
- ✓ eat whole grains;
- ✓ drink alcohol in moderation;
- ✓ restrict calories;
- ✓ exercise;
- ✓ avoid direct sun exposure;
- ✓ get vaccinated; and
- ✓ have regular check-ups.

This advice is echoed by every reputable source, including the American Cancer Society,[34] the Centers for Disease Control and Prevention,[35] and the Harvard School of Public Health,[36] among others.

The Agency for Healthcare Research and Quality (AHRQ) is an excellent resource for patients and their advocates. The AHRQ is the federal government's leading agency charged with improving the quality, safety, efficiency and effectiveness of healthcare for all Americans. The website, AHRQ.gov, offers consumer-friendly podcasts, detailing the necessary health screening needed to prevent disease.

Chapter 2

Using Reliable Resources to Manage Health

Whether we are interested in maintaining our health or learning more about our medical condition and/or proposed treatment, it is easy to become overwhelmed with the volume of available information. The following list is not intended to be all inclusive, but a good start to helpful, reliable patient information. Some sites are disease-specific, others are intended to help in disease prevention.

American Cancer Society provides information about cancer, its treatments and ongoing research, and cancer support groups for both patients and their loved ones. http://www.cancer.org/index

American Lung Association provides information about lung cancer, asthma, COPD and other lung disorders, as well as ongoing research. http://www.lung.org/

American Diabetes Association provides information about diabetes, its treatments, and ongoing research, and offers patients advice on nutrition and meal planning, fitness regimes, and lifestyle changes, and connects them with support groups in their communities. http://www.diabetes.org/

American Heart Association's HeartHub is a patient portal for information, tools and resources on heart disease and stroke. The site includes information on supplies, tools, videos, recipes, exercise tips, and expert advice for patients with heart disease and their families. http://hearthub.org/

Federal Drug Administration (FDA) provides information including the medication guide and instructions on how to buy and use drugs effectively. http://www.fda.gov/

HealthFinders provides information on health topics and provides resources for government, non-profit organizations and universities. It includes a tool for patients to stay current on required health screenings and related healthcare issues. http://www.healthfinder.gov/Default.aspx

Mayo Clinic offers extensive disease/condition information, symptoms, tests and procedures, and facts about drugs and supplements. http://www.mayoclinic.org/patient-care-and-health-information

National Institutes of Health (NIH) provides information on medical conditions, causes, symptoms, and treatments by linking to trusted websites for specific information. http://health.nih.gov/

NIH MedlinePlus. The NIH, along with the National Library of Medicine provides information about diseases, conditions, prescription drugs, and over-the-counter medicines. The site also contains wellness guidelines, tools and videos for patients of all ages. http://www.nlm.nih.gov/medlineplus/

Substance Abuse and Mental Health Services Administration (SAMHSA) provides information concerning substance abuse and mental health prevention, treatment, recovery, grants and funding opportunities, agency administrative information and contacts, places to purchase distributable documentation, and other resources. http://www.samhsa.gov/index.aspx

Chapter 3
Preparing for Medical Appointments

The Agency for Healthcare Research and Quality (AHRQ), defines quality healthcare as "doing the right thing for the right patient, at the right time, in the right way to achieve the best possible results."[37] Thus for the purpose of this discussion quality healthcare means: obtaining the healthcare services we need, when we need them, using the appropriate test or procedure, to achieve the best possible results.

Preparing for medical appointments is a critical step to obtaining quality care.   I strongly recommend adopting the following AHRQ recommendations on how to prepare for medical appointments, available online at: http://www.ahrq.gov/patients-consumers/index.html.

- ✓ Asking someone to go to your appointment with you to help you understand and remember answers to your questions;
- ✓ Creating a health history that includes your current conditions and past surgeries or illnesses and taking it with you to your appointment;
- ✓ Knowing your family's health history, such as your parents' health conditions; and
- ✓ Bringing all your medicines with you.

AHQR identifies the following as 10 Questions to ask your doctor:

1. What is the test for?
2. How many times have you done this procedure?
3. When will I get the results?
4. Why do I need this treatment?
5. Are there any alternatives?
6. What are the possible complications?
7. Which hospital is best for my needs?
8. How do you spell the name of that drug?
9. Are there any side effects?
10. Will this medicine interact with medicines that I'm already taking?

To obtain quality care, we must come to our appointments prepared, ask questions, and supplement the information with reliable resources.

Advocate's Checklist:

Actively participate in my healthcare by:

✓ *Staying healthy*
✓ *Using reliable resources to manage health*
✓ *Preparing for medical appointments*

Part III

Understanding Patient Rights

Improving patient experience requires us to understand what rights apply to each situation and how to protect those rights. In the following chapters, we discuss in detail patient rights that, in my experience, are most commonly at issue:

- ➤ HIPAA Privacy
- ➤ Billing
- ➤ Discharge
- ➤ Emergency Medical Treatment
- ➤ Durable Medical Equipment
- ➤ Medical Errors

To test your understanding of patients' rights, take the Advocate's Quiz beginning on the next page. You can find the answers by reviewing the information on the pages noted under each question.

Advocates Patients' Rights Quiz

1. My dad lives in a nursing home and complains (loudly) about the poor service and food. The nursing home administrator told me they are discharging him from the home because of his disruptive behavior. Can the home do that?

   [Nursing home residents' discharge rights are discussed on pages 108-111.]

2. I am constantly receiving fundraising mailers from the hospital where I had surgery. Is there a way I can get them to stop sending these to me?

   [Patients' right to opt out of fundraising communications is discussed on page 75.]

3. I am changing healthcare providers and asked my physician's secretary to send my records to my new physician. It's been five weeks and she still has not sent my records? How long do I have to wait?

   [Individuals' right to receive a copy of their medical records is discussed on pages 65-67.]

4. My disabled sister lives in her own home. She finally received the wheelchair Medicare promised, but the chair's battery stopped working within the first week. She is really upset. What can she do about this?

   [Consumers' rights related to durable medical equipment are discussed on pages 114-117.]

5. My wife is currently in the hospital recovering from a stroke. I just overheard the nurses say they need the bed and are going to send my wife home with me tomorrow. She is making progress slowly, but there is no way she is ready to come home. What should I do to make sure she is not discharged before she is ready?

   [A Medicare beneficiary's right to appeal a hospital discharge is discussed on pages 105-107.]

6. My neighbor asked me for advice on how to choose medical insurance. What resources are available?

   [Guidance about choosing health insurance is provided on pages 22-26.]

7. My client's medical information, including his Social Security number, was posted on the Internet by his health insurance company. When we called the insurance agent, she advised that the company is aware and intends to remove the information. What responsibility does the insurance company have to address this?

[Breach notification requirements are discussed on pages 78-79.]

8. I took my son to the emergency department because his asthma got bad. The receptionist told me it would be a long wait and I should take my child to another hospital ED an hour away. I drove to the other hospital and they treated my child, but I am very upset about the first hospital's refusal to see him. What are a patient's rights when it comes to emergency treatment?

[The Emergency Medical Treatment and Labor Act is discussed on page 113.]

Chapter 1
Knowing Our Rights

Patient rights come from many sources. Medicare and Medicaid certified healthcare providers must meet minimum standards called Conditions of Participation (CoP) or Conditions for Coverage (CfC). CoPs and CfCs, which can be found in the Code of Federal Regulations (CFR), include patient rights. The CFR contains all of the regulations issued by federal administrative agencies, such as the Department of Health and Human Services (DHHS). The CFR is available online at: http://www.ecfr.gov/cgi-bin/ECFR?page=browse

Patient rights regulations often incorporate by reference rights found elsewhere in federal and state law. Interpretive Guidelines provide surveyors with guidance that clarifies and/or explains the intent of the regulation.

Patient rights might also arise from accreditation standards. To ensure that healthcare providers meet CoPs or CfCs, CMS relies on two types of external review: *accreditation* and *certification* by State Agencies. Providers and suppliers accredited by an approved national accreditation organization (AO) may be exempt from routine surveys by State Survey Agencies. AOs have standards, including patient rights, which may mirror or exceed CMS regulations. In order to be accredited, providers must meet the standards of the AO.[38]

Patient rights also come from federal regulations such as the Patient Self-Determination Act (PSDA), Emergency Medical Treatment and Labor Act (EMTALA), Health Insurance Portability and Accountability Act of 1996 (HIPAA); and the Americans with Disabilities Act (ADA).

Patient quality care rights are the mirror image of providers' responsibilities. For instance, nursing facilities must ensure that each resident maintains the ability to perform activities of daily living (such as grooming, toileting, eating and ambulating) unless the resident's clinical condition demonstrates that loss of ability was unavoidable.[39] The resident's right to receive care necessary to maintain activities of daily living is implied in this requirement.

Patient rights also come from state laws, including laws governing licensure and certification of mental health, developmental disabilities, and older adults and children services. Patient rights found in state law may mirror or exceed patient rights found in federal law. Where there is a conflict, federal law trumps state law.

While patient rights found in state law are not detailed in this book, patients and their advocates must be familiar with their state's laws, rules and requirements.

Sometimes legal analysis is required to determine whether or not a specific patient right applies to a particular situation. For instance, some of the rights set forth in the Hospital CoPs (such as the right to give or withhold informed consent or the right to file a grievance) apply to most hospital patients.

However, some of the rights (such as the right to appeal a discharge), apply only to Medicare beneficiaries.

Whether patient rights, such as those included in EMTALA (discussed on page 113), apply to a particular situation may also depend on the facts of the case.

Because this book is intended as a general overview and not as legal advice, patients and their advocates should always seek legal counsel when clarification is needed.

The chart below identifies the federal regulation pertaining to healthcare consumer rights organized by provider type.

Healthcare Consumer Rights		
Provider Type	**Federal Regulation**	**Grievance Rights**
Ambulatory Surgical Center	42 CFR §416.50	42 CFR §416.50(d)
Durable Medical Equipment Provider	42 CFR §425.57	42 CFR §425.57(c)
End Stage Renal Disease Facility	42 CFR §494.70	42 CFR §494.80(e)
Home Health Services	42 CFR §484.10	42 CFR §484.10(b)(4) &(5)
Hospice	42 CFR §418.52	42 CFR §418.52(b)(1)(iii)
Hospital	42 CFR §482.13	42 CFR §482.13(a)(2)
Nursing Home	42 CFR §483.10	42 CFR §483.10(f)

Chapter 2
HIPAA Privacy Rights

This chapter informs patients and advocates about their privacy rights and provides guidance on what to do if problems arise. Advocates can feel confident they have the tools necessary to protect the privacy of patient information.

The Importance of Protecting Our Medical Information

The fact that the paper medical record is fast becoming a relic brings with it benefits and risks. Medical information stored and shared electronically allows:

> ➢ Healthcare providers to instantly share critical information about their patients, avoiding mistakes and unnecessary tests;
> ➢ Insurance companies to pay claims without delay; and
> ➢ Patients to view their information online to promptly receive results and ensure accuracy of their record.

Immediate sharing of electronic medical information can mean the difference between life and death. An unconscious patient brought by ambulance to the emergency department needs the treating physician to click on her electronic medical record to learn about her life-threatening allergy to penicillin. There is no time to wait for the medical records department to locate and deliver the paper chart to the physician.

The downside of the electronic medical record is the heightened risk of large scale identity theft, which is often a stepping-stone to medical billing fraud. It can occur when dishonest people working in a medical setting use patient information to submit false bills to government or private insurers.

Medical identity theft occurs when someone uses another person's name or insurance information to get medical treatment, prescription drugs or surgery. Because of medical identity theft, patients often bear the cost of increased health insurance premiums, legal fees, lost time and productivity trying to fix the problem, an inaccurate credit report, and/or out-of-pocket payments to the health plan or insurer.

The U.S. Department of Health and Human Services (HHS) Office for Civil Rights (OCR), the government agency responsible for enforcing the HIPAA Privacy Rule, reports that the primary cause of HIPAA breaches in 2010 was theft of individuals' information.[40]

A breach is the acquisition, access, use, or disclosure of protected health information (PHI) in a manner that compromises the security or privacy of that information. Among the 207 breaches that affected 500 or more individuals in 2010, 99 incidents involved theft of paper records or electronic media, together affecting approximately 2,979,121 individuals.[41]

The cost of identity theft is staggering. The National Health Care Anti-Fraud Association estimates that fraud collectively costs Americans between $70 billion and $234 billion a year.[42]

The FBI estimates that fraudulent billings to public and private healthcare programs account for between 3 and 10 percent of total healthcare expenditures.[43]

Identity theft is not the only threat to patient privacy. Carelessness by providers such as physician offices, hospitals, pharmacies and insurance companies can threaten the privacy of patient information.

According to the OCR, providers' most common HIPAA violations are:

1. impermissible uses and disclosures of protected health information;
2. lack of safeguards for protected health information;
3. lack of patient access to their protected health information;
4. uses or disclosures of more than the minimum necessary protected health information; and
5. failure to provide individuals with a Notice of Privacy Practices.[44]

Examples of violations identified by the OCR include:[45]

> A radiology practice that interpreted a hospital patient's imaging tests submitted a worker's compensation claim to the patient's employer. The claim included the patient's test results. However, the patient was not covered by worker's compensation and had not identified worker's compensation as responsible for payment.

> A staff member of a medical practice discussed HIV testing procedures with a patient in the waiting room, thereby disclosing protected health information to several other individuals.

> After treating a patient who was injured in an accident, the hospital released patient information, including copies of the patient's skull x-ray and a description of the complainant's medical condition, to the local media. The local newspaper then featured on its front-page the individual's x-ray and an article that included the date of the accident, the location of the accident, the patient's gender, a description of the patient's medical condition, and numerous quotes from the hospital about the injury.

> A hospital employee did not observe minimum necessary requirements when she left a telephone message with the daughter of a patient detailing both her medical condition and treatment plan.

Patients pay a high price when their information is used or disclosed without a business reason. Information lost or placed in the wrong patient chart may delay or negatively impact care.

Information disclosed to the wrong place may cause embarrassment, discrimination or denial of insurance.

Whether in paper or electronic format, healthcare providers must protect the privacy of an individual's medical information. Protecting patient privacy is a joint effort between the covered entity, the government and the individual.

Patients and their advocates play a critical role protecting the privacy of individual health information. By knowing their rights, monitoring the accuracy of their medical records, and watching for signs of medical identity theft, patients can avoid or mitigate harm caused by mistakes or fraud.

Understanding HIPAA

In 1996, Congress passed the Health Insurance Portability and Accountability Act of 1996 (HIPAA) which, among other things, required the U.S. Department of Health & Human Services (HHS) to issue patient privacy protections. The HIPAA Privacy Rule (hereafter "the Privacy Rule"), which took effect on April 14, 2003, ensures a national minimum standard of privacy by limiting the ways that health plans, pharmacies, hospitals and other covered entities can use or disclose patients' protected health information (PHI), whether it is on paper, in computers or communicated verbally.

The Privacy Rule recognizes the importance of the free flow of PHI for safe and effective delivery of healthcare, while setting limits to what healthcare providers can do with that information. The Privacy Rule mandates the implementation of appropriate safeguards to protect the privacy of PHI and sets limits and conditions on the uses and disclosures of such information without patient authorization.

Use means the sharing, employment, application, utilization, examination, or analysis of PHI *within* an entity that maintains such information. *Disclosure* means the release, transfer, provision of, access to, or divulging in any manner of PHI *outside* the entity holding the information.[46]

In February 2003, HHS published a final Security Rule, setting national standards for protecting the confidentiality, integrity, and availability of electronic PHI.

Compliance with the Security Rule was required by April 20, 2005 (April 20, 2006 for small health plans).

On October 29, 2009, HHS published the HITECH Act Enforcement Interim Final Rule that increased the penalties for HIPAA violations and gave the OCR additional enforcement authority.

As indicated in the chart below, the financial penalties for violating the Privacy and Security Rules increase according to a covered entity's awareness of and disregard for its responsibilities.

Allowable Penalties Under HITECH for Violations of HIPAA

Type of Offense	Minimum Penalty Per Violation	Aggregate Annual Penalty Cap
No actual or reasonable knowledge of violation	$100	$25,000
Reasonable knowledge of violation	$1,000	$100,000
Willful neglect with correction	$10,000	$250,000
Willful neglect without correction	$50,000	$1,500,000

The HITECH Act also gave State Attorneys General the authority to bring civil actions and obtain damages on behalf of state residents for violations of the HIPAA Privacy and Security Rules.

On January 25, 2013, HHS published the HITECH Final Rule[47] that, among other things, amended the HIPAA Privacy and Security Rules and adopted the majority of provisions of the HITECH Act Enforcement Interim Rule.[48] Covered entities had to comply with the HITECH Final Rule by September 23, 2013.

The following discussion focuses on federal regulations, specifically the Privacy Rule. Most states have their own privacy laws, which may mirror or be stricter than the Privacy Rule. Patient and advocates must reference their state laws when determining rights and responsibilities.

How the Privacy Rule Protects Patient Information

While almost everyone has heard of "HIPAA," there is much confusion about this complicated Privacy Rule.

In order to protect their privacy rights, patients and advocates must understand when the Privacy Rule applies to a particular situation and when it does not.

Before boldly proclaiming "My HIPAA rights have been violated!" patients and their advocates need to know the answers to:

1. Who must follow the Privacy Rule?
2. What information does the Privacy Rule protect?
3. How does the Privacy Rule permit covered entities to use and disclose PHI?
4. What are our privacy rights?

The four-part analysis is discussed on the following pages.

1. Who must follow the Privacy Rule?

Individuals and entities required to comply with the Privacy Rule are called *covered entities*. They include:

Health Plans, including health insurance companies, Health Maintenance Organizations (HMOs), company health plans, and certain government programs that pay for healthcare, such as Medicare and Medicaid.

Most Healthcare Providers, including those that conduct certain business electronically (such as electronically billing health insurance), most doctors, clinics, hospitals, psychologists, chiropractors, nursing homes, pharmacies, and dentists.

Healthcare Clearinghouses, defined as entities that process nonstandard health information they receive from another entity into a standard (i.e., standard electronic format or data content), or vice versa.

A covered entity's *business associate* (an individual or entity that receives patient information to carry out healthcare activities such as billing or record storage) is directly liable for compliance with certain provisions of the Privacy and Security Rules.

Under the HITECH Final Rule, a business associate's subcontractor who receives patient information is also required to comply with certain provisions of the Privacy and Security Rules.[49]

Many organizations such as life insurers, workers' compensation carriers, many state agencies and law enforcement agencies, are not required to follow the Privacy Rule.

2. What information does the Privacy Rule protect?

The Privacy Rule protects *Protected Health Information*, which is referred to as "PHI." PHI includes any information created or received by a covered entity relating to:

➤ the past, present or future physical or mental health or condition of a patient; or

➤ payment for the provision of healthcare to a patient that is transmitted or maintained in any form or medium.

PHI contains identifiers for which there is a reasonable basis to believe the information can be used to identify a patient.

Examples of PHI include:

> information entered into patient medical records by doctors, nurses, and other healthcare providers;
> conversations between doctors and nurses regarding the care or treatment of patients;
> information about individuals contained in the health insurer's computer system;
> billing information about individuals; and
> most other health information about individuals held by covered entities.

Information NOT protected under the Privacy Rule includes:

> Employment Records. The Privacy Rule does not protect an individual's employment records, even if the information in those records is health-related. If an individual works for a health plan or covered healthcare provider, the Privacy Rule does not apply to the individual's employment records. However, the Privacy Rule does protect an individual's medical or health plan records if that individual is a patient of the provider or a member of the health plan.
> De-identified Information. PHI that has been stripped of any patient identifiers (such as name, medical record number, Social Security number, date of birth, etc.) is not PHI.[50]
> Individually identifiable health information of persons who have been deceased for more than 50 years.

3. How does the Privacy Rule permit covered entities to use and disclose PHI?

The Privacy Rule balances the need for the free flow of patient information with an individual's right to privacy. Therefore, the Privacy Rule allows the use or disclosure of PHI without authorization in some instances and, at other times, requires the provider to obtain authorization from the patient in advance of certain uses or disclosures. Patients and their advocates must understand when an authorization is and is not required.

Healthcare providers may use or disclose PHI *without* the patient's authorization in the following situations:

> ➤ Treatment. Doctors, nurses, hospitals, laboratory technicians, and other healthcare providers may use or disclose PHI, such as X-rays, laboratory and pathology reports, diagnoses, and other medical information for treatment purposes without the patient's authorization. This includes sharing information to consult with other providers (including providers who are not covered entities) and to treat or refer the patient.

> ➤ Payment. Covered entities may send a patient's PHI to the insurance company in order to collect payment.

> ➤ Operations. Covered entities may use or disclose PHI for quality assurance, peer review, and business planning activities.

> ➢ Required reporting to public health agencies;

> ➢ When requested or sought by law enforcement under certain circumstancees;

> ➢ Certain emergency situations; and

> ➢ Research studies that have obtained an authorization waiver from the Institutional Review Board.

In instances other than those listed above, a covered entity must obtain a valid authorization from the individual before using or disclosing PHI. The Privacy Rule specifically requires authorization before using or disclosing:

> ➢ psychotherapy notes;[51]

> ➢ PHI for the purpose of marketing;[52] or

> ➢ PHI for sale.[53]

If a covered entity obtains a valid authorization, its use or disclosure of PHI must be consistent with that authorization.

To ensure appropriate use and disclosure of PHI, covered entities must:

- ➢ Put in place safeguards to protect individuals' health information;
- ➢ Reasonably limit uses and disclosures to the minimum necessary to accomplish their intended purpose;
- ➢ Have contracts (called business associate agreements) in place with their contractors and others ensuring that they use and disclose individuals' health information properly and safeguard it appropriately; and
- ➢ Have procedures in place to limit who can view and access individuals' health information, as well as conduct training programs for employees about how to protect individuals' health information.

The Privacy Rule specially protects certain information, including genetic information,[54] psychotherapy notes,[55] and addiction diagnosis and treatment.[56] Many states mirror these protections or provide additional protection. Patients and their advocates should refer to their state's privacy laws.

4. What are our HIPAA Privacy Rights?

Providers and health insurers who are required to follow the HIPAA Privacy Rule must comply with individuals' right to:

- ➤ Receive a Notice of Privacy Practices;
- ➤ Copy and inspect their PHI;
- ➤ Request amendments to their PHI;
- ➤ Request an accounting of disclosures of their PHI;
- ➤ Restrict the use and disclosure of their PHI;
- ➤ Request alternative means of communicating their PHI;
- ➤ Opt out of fundraising communications;
- ➤ Opt out of the facility directory;
- ➤ Restrict use of PHI for marketing purposes; and
- ➤ Receive notice of a breach of unsecured PHI.

These rights are discussed on the following pages.

Receiving a Notice of Privacy Practices[57]

The Privacy Rule requires covered entities to provide individuals with a Notice of Privacy Practices (NPP), explaining their privacy rights.[58] In order to protect one's HIPAA privacy rights, advocates should review the NPP and ask for an explanation if needed.

The NPP must be written in plain language and describe:

> - how the covered entity may use and disclose PHI about an individual;
> - the covered entity's legal duties with respect to the information, including a statement that the covered entity is required by law to maintain the privacy of PHI;
> - when the covered entity must obtain an individual's authorization prior to using or disclosing PHI, including for marketing purposes or selling PHI;
> - individuals' rights with respect to their PHI, including the right to opt out of fundraising communications and receive notice of a breach of the individual's PHI;
> - how to exercise their rights, including filing a complaint with the covered entity and/or the OCR; and
> - the name and contact information of the person individuals can contact for further information about the covered entity's privacy policies or to make a complaint.

Copying and Inspecting Your Medical Records[59]

Except in certain circumstances, individuals have the right to review and obtain a copy of their PHI in a covered entity's designated record set. The *designated record set* is that group of records maintained by or for a covered entity that is used, in whole or part, to make decisions about individuals; or a provider's medical and billing records about individuals, or a health plan's enrollment, payment, claims adjudication, and case or medical management record systems.

The HITECH Final Rule gives individuals the right to request the healthcare provider furnish their electronic PHI in an electronic format.

Individuals do not have the right to access psychotherapy notes or information compiled for legal proceedings.

Covered entities may deny access to medical records in certain specified situations, such as when a healthcare professional believes access could cause harm to the individual or another.

In those situations, the covered entity must give the individual the right to have such denials reviewed by a licensed healthcare professional.

A provider cannot deny individuals a copy of their records because they have not paid for the services received.

The covered entity must act on a request for access no later than 30 days after receipt of the request. If the covered entity is unable to act on the request within 30 days, it may extend the time frame only once for an additional 30 days, if it provides the patient with a written statement of the reason for the delay and the date it will complete its action on the request.

Covered entities may impose reasonable, cost-based fees for copying and postage. Cost must be limited to:

> ➢ labor for copying, whether in paper or electronic form. Labor can include technically trained staff that performs functions of creation, compilation, extraction, scanning, or burning;
> ➢ supplies (paper or electronic media);
> ➢ postage; and
> ➢ an explanation if requested by the individual.

The healthcare provider may not charge a retrieval fee, or include costs to pay for infrastructure or overhead.

Most states have laws governing when and how much providers may charge for medical records. Patients and their advocates should be aware of their state's laws regarding medical record fees.

Requesting Changes to Your Medical Records[60]

The Privacy Rule gives individuals the right to have covered entities amend their PHI in a designated record set when that information is inaccurate or incomplete.

As more and more patients have access to their electronic health record, they are seeing things in their record they want removed or changed. If the objectionable information is inaccurate or incomplete, the healthcare provider must amend the record. For example, if a 40-year old female patient reads in her record that she has had prostate cancer, she has a right to (and certainly should) request the amendment of the error.

Occasionally the amendment request is not so simple. A patient may object to terminology he or she finds offensive.

For instance, a patient may object to being described as "obese." The test is whether the note is accurate and complete. If the patient's Body Mass Index (BMI) is 30 or greater, the term "obese," though viewed by the patient as offensive, is medically accurate and complete and not subject to amendment.

If a covered entity agrees to amend the record, it must advise the patient and amend the record accordingly. Additionally, the covered entity must make reasonable efforts to provide the amendment to persons whom the individual has identified as needing it and to persons that the covered entity knows might rely on the information to the individual's detriment.

If the covered entity denies the amendment request, it must provide the individual with a written denial and allow the individual to submit a statement of disagreement for inclusion in the record.

In lieu of a statement of disagreement, the individual may request that the covered entity provide the individual's request for amendment and the denial with any future disclosures of the PHI in question.

The Privacy Rule details the process for requesting and responding to a request for amendment. A covered entity must amend PHI in its designated record set upon receipt of notice to amend from another covered entity.

The covered entity must act on the request for amendment no later than 60 days after receipt of the request. If the covered entity is unable to act on the amendment within 60 days, it may extend the time frame only once for an additional 30 days, if it provides the patient a written statement of the reason for the delay and the date it will complete its action on the request.

Requesting an Accounting of Disclosures[61]

Individuals have a right to an accounting of the disclosures of their PHI by a covered entity or the covered entity's business associates. The maximum disclosure accounting period is the six years immediately preceding the accounting request.

The Privacy Rule does not require accounting for disclosures:

- of treatment, payment, or healthcare operations;
- to the individual or the individual's personal representative;
- for notification of or to persons involved in an individual's healthcare or payment for healthcare, for disaster relief, or for facility directories;
- pursuant to an authorization;
- of a limited data set;
- for national security or intelligence purposes;
- to correctional institutions or law enforcement officials for certain purposes regarding inmates or individuals in lawful custody; or
- incident to otherwise permitted or required uses or disclosures.

The covered entity must temporarily suspend the inclusion of an accounting for disclosures to health oversight agencies and law enforcement officials if the covered entity receives a written notice that an accounting would likely impede their activities.

The covered entity must act on the request no later than 60 days after receipt of the request.

If the covered entity is unable to act on the request within 60 days, it may extend the time frame only once for an additional 30 days, if it provides the patient a written statement of the reason for the delay and the date it will complete its action on the request.

Restricting Use and Disclosure of Your Medical Information[62]

Patients have the right to request a healthcare provider restrict the use or disclosure of their PHI. While patients may *request* the restriction, healthcare providers must only agree to an individual's request if the following conditions are met:

> ➤ the disclosure is to the individual's health plan for the purpose of collecting payment, or healthcare operations such as quality review;
> ➤ the disclosure to the health plan is not required by law; and
> ➤ the individual, or person (other than the health plan) on behalf of the individual, has paid the covered entity in full.

For instance, an individual undergoing genetic testing may wish to pay out-of-pocket and block the information from going to his or her insurance company. If the three conditions are met, in most cases, the covered entity must grant the exception.

Be advised when a healthcare provider grants the restriction request, it is not the provider's responsibility to notify downstream providers, such as pharmacies or specialists, of the restriction request.

Instead, it is the responsibility of the individual to notify downstream providers.

For example, a patient sees his primary care physician (PCP) and requests a restriction on tests being administered to determine if he has HIV or other sexually transmitted diseases. If, after conducting the tests, the PCP refers the patient to an infectious disease specialist, it is the patient's obligation to request a restriction from that specialist if he wishes to pay out-of-pocket rather than have his health insurance billed for the visit.

Likewise, the patient, not the provider, must notify the pharmacist if the patient wishes to pay out-of-pocket for his medication and not have his insurance company billed.

Requesting Alternative Means of Communicating Your Medical Information[63]

A covered healthcare provider must accommodate reasonable requests by individuals to receive communications of medical information from the covered healthcare provider by alternative means or at alternative locations.

For example, an individual may request that the provider communicate with the individual through a specified address or phone number. Similarly, an individual may request that the provider send communications in a closed envelope rather than a postcard.

Prior to accommodating an individual's request for alternative means of communicating, a covered entity may require that the individual provide information as to how payment will be handled and an alternative address or other method of contact.

Opting Out of Fundraising Communications[64]

In certain circumstances, a covered entity may use or disclose PHI to its institutionally-related foundation or another business for the purpose of raising funds without obtaining patient authorization.   A covered entity is permitted to use or disclose a patient's demographic information (including name, age, gender, date of birth, address, and other contact information), dates of healthcare provided to an individual, department of service, treating physician, outcome information; and health insurance status. A covered entity may not use treatment or diagnosis information to fundraise without patient authorization.

Every fundraising communication must include a notice informing the individual of the right to opt out of future solicitations. The covered entity must provide an easy way for individuals to opt out, such as toll-free number or email address. Requiring the individual to write a letter in order to opt out is not permitted under the Privacy Rule.

Opting Out of the Facility Directory[65]

A healthcare provider has the right to use or disclose certain patient information for the facility's directory unless the patient objects. To create the directory, the provider may use an individual's name, location in the healthcare facility, the individual's general condition (but not specific medical information); and the individual's religious affiliation. The provider may share this information with members of the clergy and, except for religious affiliation, other persons who ask for the patient by name.

Except in certain emergencies, the healthcare provider must inform the patient about the directory and allow the patient to opt out.

Restricting Use of Your Medical Information for Marketing Purposes[66]

The Privacy Rule requires a covered entity to obtain individuals' authorization prior to using their PHI for marketing purposes. To fully understand an individual's right to restrict the use of PHI for marketing, patients and their advocates must know how the Privacy Rule defines _marketing_.

Marketing is "a communication about a product or service that encourages recipients of the communication to purchase or use the product or service." The following are exceptions to the definition of "marketing" and a covered entity does not need patient authorization to perform them.

➢ Provide drug refill reminders;
➢ Describe a health-related product or service that is provided by, or included in the provider's plan of benefits; and
➢ Case management or care coordination.

Receiving Notice of a Breach of Your Medical Information[67]

A breach is an impermissible use or disclosure under the Privacy Rule that compromises the security or privacy of PHI.

Covered entities must notify affected individuals following the discovery of a breach of unsecured PHI. Covered entities must provide this individual notice in written form by first-class mail, or alternatively, by email if the affected individual has agreed to receive such notices electronically. The breach notification, which must be provided no later than 60 days following the discovery of a breach, must include:

➢ a description of the breach;
➢ a description of the types of information involved in the breach;
➢ the steps affected individuals should take to protect themselves from potential harm;
➢ a brief description of what the covered entity is doing to investigate the breach, mitigate the harm, and prevent further breaches; and
➢ the covered entity's contact information.

The law also requires a covered entity to notify the Secretary of the U.S. Department of Health and Human Services (HHS). If a breach affects more than 500 residents of a state or jurisdiction, the covered entity must also notify prominent media outlets serving the state or jurisdiction.

Most Commonly Asked HIPAA Questions

The following questions and answers are from the HHS OCR website: http://www.hhs.gov/ocr/privacy/hipaa/understanding/consumers/index.html.

Does my physician need my authorization to send my medical records to the specialist I am seeing?

No. The Privacy Rule permits a healthcare provider to disclose PHI without the individual's authorization to another healthcare provider for that provider's treatment of the individual.

Is my healthcare provider permitted to send my medical information to the collection agency without my authorization?

Yes. The Privacy Rule permits covered entities to use the services of debt collection agencies to collect payment. The provider must only send the information necessary to collect payment. If your healthcare provider sent your entire medical chart to the collection agency, it is likely a HIPAA violation.

May my healthcare provider discuss my medical information with my friends or family without my authorization?

As long as you do not object, the Privacy Rule allows your healthcare provider to share or discuss your health information with your family, friends, or others if they are involved in your care or payment for your care.

Your provider may ask your permission, may tell you he or she plans to discuss the information and give you an opportunity to object, or may decide, using his or her professional judgment, that you do not object. In any of these cases, your healthcare provider may discuss only the information that the person involved needs to know about your care or payment for your care. For example, the Privacy Rule:

➢ allows your physician to talk with your friend who is driving you home from the hospital about keeping your foot raised during the ride home.

➢ allows the nurse to discuss your medications with your health aide who accompanied you to your appointment.

➢ does not permit the doctor to discuss your condition with your mother-in-law if you told her not to.

➢ does not permit the nurse to discuss your past medical history with your spouse if it is unrelated to your current condition.

I was being treated in the Emergency Department and could hear the doctor in the next room talking to a patient about his diagnosis. Isn't that a violation of HIPAA?

The Privacy Rule does not require providers to soundproof rooms or have individual patient rooms. However, providers are required to use reasonable safeguards, such as lowering their voices when discussing patient information. Providers may not discuss patient information in a public area such as a waiting room or hospital cafeteria where passersby could easily hear.

My physician's office leaves messages on my answering machine to let me know about my next appointment. Is that permissible under HIPAA?

The Privacy Rule allows healthcare providers to communicate with patients at their homes, whether through the mail or phone. Providers may leave messages for their patients, but must use reasonable safeguards, such as limiting the amount and type of information left on the message machine. If you request that your provider communicate with you in a certain way, the Privacy Rule requires the provider to comply with your wishes.

While visiting a friend at the hospital, I walked by the nurses' station located in the middle of patient traffic and saw medical records spread out for all to see. Is this a HIPAA violation?

The Privacy Rule requires covered entities like hospitals to use reasonable safeguards to protect patient privacy. Providers may not keep patient information in an area where visitors could easily see. Charts should be stored in a secure location such as behind the nurses' station.

Five Steps to Protecting Your Medical Information

In order to protect one's medical information, patients and their advocates must be proactive. The first step, *know your privacy rights*, is based on the adage "Knowledge is power." It is only possible to protect your privacy rights if you know what they are. The second step, *recognize warning signs*, requires patients to monitor their health information in order to identity potential issues. Third, when issues or concerns regarding medical information arise, patients have the right to *hold providers accountable*. While most providers want to resolve patient concerns, it may be necessary to take the fourth step and *go up the chain of command*. The final step, *keep detailed records*, is necessary to track progress resolving questions or concerns.

Each of these steps is discussed in detail on the following pages.

Step 1: Know Your Privacy Rights

When providers are aware that you know your rights, you are one step closer to resolving the issue. There is a big difference between proclaiming, "You people violated my HIPAA rights," and "Under the Privacy Rule, you have 30 days to provide me my medical records. It is day 27 and I want to resolve this without calling the Office for Civil Rights." Using the second approach, you are likely to receive your medical records without escalation.

Knowing your rights begins with reading the Notice of Privacy Practices (NPP) and asking questions if you need clarification. The NPP is a document worth understanding and keeping for future reference. The NPP spells out your privacy rights and the purposes for which the covered entity may use and disclose your PHI.

Many of the privacy rights include a time frame within which providers must comply.

For instance, you have the right to receive, and the provider has a duty to provide, a copy of your medical record within 30 days, with a possible 30-day extension following a written notice.

Likewise, you have the right to request an amendment of inaccurate information contained in your medical record.

The covered entity must respond to your request within 60 days with a possible 30-day extension, when a written notice has been provided.

A covered entity that ignores its responsibilities under the Privacy Rule is subject to potential financial penalties. By understanding your rights and the covered entity's responsibilities, you are in the best position to hold providers accountable.

Step 2: Recognize Warning Signs

To protect yourself from harm caused by inappropriate use or disclosure of PHI, familiarize yourself with the signs of wrongdoing. Indications that you may be a victim of medical identity theft include:

- a bill for medical services you did not receive;
- a call from a debt collector about a medical debt you do not owe;
- medical collection notices on your credit report that you do not recognize;
- a notice from your health plan saying you reached your benefit limit, when you know you did not;
- a denial of insurance because your medical records show a condition you do not have; and/or
- information in your medical record that does not pertain to you.[68]

To recognize signs of potential trouble you must regularly read the Explanation of Benefits (EOB) statement or Medicare Summary Notice that your health plan sends after treatment. Check the name of the provider, the date of service, and the service provided. If the claims do not match the care you received, contact your health plan and report the problem.

Keeping an eye on your medical information is becoming easier as an increasing number of healthcare providers offer patients online access to their information. If this option is available, take advantage of it and review your medical information regularly.

If online access to medical information is not available, obtain a copy of your medical record for review.

If the medical record contains incomplete or inaccurate information, the cause may be provider error or medical identity theft. In either case, be sure to exercise your right to request an amendment as discussed on pages 67-69.

The Federal Bureau of Investigation (FBI) provides the following tips to protect oneself from healthcare fraud:

> ➤ Protect your health insurance information card like you would a credit card.
> ➤ Beware of free services—they may be too good to be true.
> ➤ Review your medical bills, such as your "Explanation of Benefits," after receiving healthcare services. Check the dates and services to ensure you received what you are being billed for.
> ➤ If you suspect healthcare fraud, contact your insurance company, your local FBI field office and/or the HHS Office of Inspector General (OIG).[69]

Patients and their advocates are in the best position to monitor the accuracy of their medical records and recognize signs of provider error, healthcare fraud, or identity theft. Timely identification of a potential issue may reduce the risk of harm. For instance, if a patient identifies inaccurate information in the medical record, the patient can pursue an amendment before the erroneous information is disclosed to other clinicians. If a patient suspects identity theft, notifying authorities and obtaining credit monitoring may mitigate harm done to one's personal finances. Being proactive is the best way to protect patient privacy.

Step 3: Hold Providers Accountable

The OCR expects covered entities to resolve privacy concerns in a timely manner and document all privacy concerns received, as well as the outcome of the investigation.[70]   Patients and their advocates who raise privacy concerns should expect a prompt and meaningful response to those matters.

The Privacy Rule requires covered entities to designate a contact person to receive complaints about privacy and provide information about the covered entity's NPP.[71]

While not required, patients and their representatives should contact the provider's privacy designee as a first step to resolving the concern. The Privacy Rule requires covered entities to have written policies and procedures to ensure compliance with the Privacy Rule and apply sanctions to those who violate those policies.[72] The covered entity's designee will know the policies and procedures and the regulatory consequences for failing to follow them.

Patients may be hesitant to mention privacy concerns for fear of upsetting their healthcare providers. Rest assured, the Privacy Rule prohibits covered entities from intimidating, threatening, coercing, discriminating against, or taking other retaliatory action against any individuals for exercising their privacy rights.[73]

Step 4: Go Up the Chain of Command

Most privacy concerns will be resolved at the level of the covered entity. However, in the event that the covered entity is not responsive, you may wish to file a complaint with the OCR.

A notable example of failing to respond to both the patients' request for their medical records and the government's request for response occurred in 2011. The OCR fined Cignet Health System $4.3 million dollars for Privacy Rule violations. The OCR assessed $1.3 million dollars of that penalty for denying 41 patients the right to access their medical records. The remaining civil monetary penalties related to the health system's failure to respond to the OCR inquiries about the patients' concerns.[74]

If your concern involves identity theft, you may also file a complaint with the Federal Trade Commission (FTC) Bureau of Consumer Protection via its website: http://business.ftc.gov.

To combat identity theft, the FTC implemented the Red Flags Rule,[75] which requires financial institutions and creditors to implement a program to detect, prevent and mitigate identity theft in connection with new and existing accounts.

The Red Flags Rule applies to hospitals, clinics and other healthcare organizations if the organizations meet the Rule's definition of "creditor" and if the organizations offer or maintain "covered accounts."

Individuals do not have a right to sue under the federal Privacy Rules, however State Attorneys General may file a claim on behalf of constituents whose privacy rights have been violated.

Many states have privacy laws under which an individual has the right to file a claim. Patients and their advocates must understand their state's privacy laws in order to determine available legal options.

Step 5: Keep Detailed Records

Resolving a privacy request or concern can require significant effort. In order to track what steps you have taken, keep a detailed record of the issue, to whom you spoke, what was discussed, and the date of the conversation. Be certain to ask the individuals' names and note their contact information (such as a phone number or email address). At the end of the conversation, thank the individual and ask if you may follow up with them if the issue remains unresolved.

As previously discussed, many of the privacy rights require covered entities to respond within a specified number of days. Keeping track of the time frame allows you to check the progress of your request.

Although not required, you may wish to send your request for amendment of your medical record by certified mail, and ask for a return receipt so you have a record of what the plan or provider received. Keep copies of all letters and documents you send and receive pertaining to your concern.

In the event that you must escalate your concern, having a detailed account of what steps you have taken in your attempt to resolve the issue may prove invaluable.

Chapter 3
Billing Rights

The most common (and valid) billing complaints I hear from patients are: healthcare costs are out of control; my bill is inaccurate; and my insurance company wrongly denied my claims.

If you think healthcare costs are out of control, you are correct. In a Time Magazine Special Report "Bitter Pill: Why Medical Bills are Killing Us,"[76] author Steven Brill examines the cost of medical care in America. He concludes there is no rhyme or reason to what healthcare providers charge patients and their insurance, and that "outrageous pricing and egregious profits are destroying our health care."

If you think your medical bill is inaccurate, you are probably right. Medical Billing Advocates of America (ABAA), a national association that assists consumers with their medical bills, advises that eight out of ten hospital bills its members scrutinize contain errors.[77]

If you think your insurance company was wrong to deny your claim, you are likely correct.

A 2012 study by the American Medical Association (AMA) found that, while billing accuracy has improved, one in ten bills paid by private health insurance have errors.

The AMA estimates that if insurers consistently paid claims correctly there would be $7 billion in health system savings due to a reduction in unnecessary administrative work to reconcile errors.[78]

Government insurance also has a high rate of incorrect denials. In 2010 Medicare denied one in ten claims. Medicare beneficiaries filed a complaint or appealed 20% of those denied claims, and half of those denials were reversed.[79]

To avoid paying inaccurate medical bills or receiving inappropriate denials of your medical claims, I recommend following these steps:

1. Give your providers accurate billing information;
2. Know what your insurance plan covers;
3. Understand your billing rights;
4. Be aware of the most common billing errors;
5. Examine every bill every time;
6. Address billing concerns immediately;
7. Appeal insurance denials; and
8. Keep excellent records.

1. Give your providers accurate billing information.

Each time you visit your physician's office, hospital, urgent care, outpatient lab or radiology department, or any other service provider, confirm that they have your current name, address, and insurance information. Do not assume that the updated information you give to one provider will transfer to other providers, even within that same system. Wrong information may result in an insurance claim denial, or your medical bills going to the wrong address.

2. Know what your insurance plan covers.

Review your insurance benefits or contact your insurance provider to determine what your policy will pay and what out-of-pocket expenses you might incur.

Patients covered by government insurance programs such as Medicare and Medicaid are better protected from uncontrolled medical costs than are patients with private insurance or no insurance. The government limits what it will pay providers and prohibits balance billing (discussed on page 98). For those of us covered by private insurance, we can avoid healthcare sticker shock by ensuring that every healthcare provider and service we use is on our insurance plan network.

Self-pay patients are the most vulnerable to back-breaking healthcare bills and should attempt to obtain some form of healthcare coverage or financial assistance prior to seeking non-emergent services.

3. Understand your billing rights.

Your healthcare billing rights depend on (1) what type of insurance you have (employer-based, government, or individual coverage); (2) from what type of healthcare provider you receive treatment or services; and (3) your state's laws.

Much of the following discussion focuses on Medicare beneficiaries' billing rights, which is dictated by federal regulation. It is essential that patients and their advocates understand the laws and rules of their state. A good place to start is your state's Department of Insurance.

Medicare beneficiary billing rights

Medicare beneficiaries have special billing protections. *First*, they have the right to know what their plan covers and can obtain that information from the Medicare.gov website:

http://www.medicare.gov/what-medicare-covers/part-a/what-part-a-covers.html.

Second, Medicare beneficiaries have the right to receive a notice of non-coverage. A Medicare beneficiary might complain "Medicare refuses to pay for my medical procedure claiming it does not cover those services. Shouldn't the doctor and hospital have informed me Medicare would not cover? Had I known, I would not have undergone the procedure."

Medicare certified healthcare providers (hospitals, independent laboratories, physicians, practitioners, and suppliers) must give Medicare beneficiaries (enrolled in Original Medicare) an Advance Beneficiary Notice of Non-coverage (ABN). The provider must give the beneficiary the ABN before services are rendered when the provider believes Medicare will not pay for some or all of the items or services because they are not reasonable and necessary under Medicare Program standards. ABNs are not required for care that is excluded by statute or for services for which no Medicare benefit category exists.

If the provider does not deliver a valid ABN to the beneficiary when required, the provider may not bill the beneficiary for the service.[80]

Third, Medicare beneficiaries have the right to receive notice of hospital-based outpatient billing charges.

A Medicare beneficiary might complain "I saw a physician and received two charges--one for the doctor and one for the facility. When I called the number on the billing statement to complain, I was told I have to pay since I chose to go to a 'hospital-based outpatient provider.' What does that mean and do I have to pay?"

"Hospital-based outpatient" refers to the billing process for services rendered in a hospital outpatient clinic or location. Patients may potentially receive two charges on their bill for services provided within a hospital-based outpatient setting. One charge (including copay and deductible) represents the facility or hospital charge and one charge (including copay and deductible) represents the professional or physician fee. Additionally, some lab tests drawn at freestanding clinics may be sent to a hospital or other facility for processing and also show a hospital outpatient lab charge.

Depending on their particular insurance coverage, patients might pay more for certain outpatient services and procedures at hospital outpatient locations.

Medicare beneficiaries are specially protected when it comes to outpatient billing.

Before delivering services, hospital-based outpatient facilities must provide written notice to Medicare beneficiaries of their potential financial liability. The notice must include an explanation that the beneficiary will incur a coinsurance liability to the hospital that the patient would not incur if the facility were not hospital-based.

The notice must also include an estimate based on typical or average charges for visits to the facility, and a statement that the patient's actual liability will depend upon the actual services furnished by the hospital.[81]

Fourth, Medicare patients have the right to file a formal grievance regarding billing concerns with the hospital. Medicare billing complaints are considered grievances and subject to the hospital patient grievance regulation.[82]

Balance billing

Balance billing occurs when physicians or other providers that are not contracted with your insurance plan bill you for the difference between the amount the provider or facility bills and the amount your health plan pays them.

Balance billing is prohibited when you have:

> ➢ Medicare and your provider accepts Medicare assignment;[83]
> ➢ Medicaid and your provider has an agreement with Medicaid;[84] or
> ➢ a health plan with whom your provider has a contract and is billing more than that contract allows.[85]

To avoid balance billing surprise, you should find out in advance of treatment whether the provider, including all facility-based providers and services, contracts with your insurance plan. If not, obtain in writing how much you will have to pay out-of-pocket for that service.

You may be able to prevent balance billing by asking that a contracted provider be assigned to your care. In certain circumstances, this option may not be available to you. For example, a hospital might staff its emergency department with a group of doctors who are not in your network.

4. Be aware of the most common billing errors.

The most common billing errors include charging for treatment or service not provided; upcoding; and unbundling services. These errors are discussed in detail below.

Charging for treatment or services not provided

If your providers cannot produce evidence that a particular treatment or service was given, they may not bill you or your insurance.

Consumer Reports suggests scrutinizing all room-and-board charges to make sure you are not inappropriately charged a full-day stay. "Many plans do not allow hospitals to charge you for your discharge day, although hospitals frequently do," the report notes. "If you went to an emergency room but weren't admitted until after midnight, you shouldn't be charged for the previous day."[86]

Medical Billing Advocates of America warns patient that they should not be billed at a private room rate when a semi-private room is not available or not requested by the patient or physician.[87]

A doctor's order is required for certain tests and procedures. The bill must reflect only those tests that were conducted in accordance with the doctor's order.

Upcoding

In order to bill a patient's insurance, the provider must assign a code to the service that reflects the patient's diagnosis and level of service received. Because reimbursement is greater for higher levels of service, an unscrupulous provider might "upcode" (use a billing code that provides a higher reimbursement rate than the billing code that actually reflects the service provided to the patient) in order to increase payment. Sometimes upcoding is caused by a clerical error. Be sure to check every billing statement and verify that the services listed were actually received.

Unbundling services

Both government and private insurers require certain tests to be "bundled" or grouped into one payment. For example, Medicare requires "all services integral to accomplishing a procedure" to be bundled. Bundled codes may not be billed separately and cannot be charged to the patient.

Contact your insurance company if you have questions whether certain fees should be bundled or may be charged separately.

5. Examine every bill every time.

Examining every bill every time is no small task. If you have been in the hospital, you may receive separate bills from the hospital (such as pharmacy, radiology, and lab charges), physicians who provided care to you during your stay, or specialists who interpreted tests results.

Compare every bill you receive from your healthcare providers with the Explanation of Benefits (EOB) statement you receive from your insurance company or the summary notice from Medicare. These statements will explain the amount:

> ➢ your providers are charging for your treatment;
> ➢ your health plan paid; and
> ➢ you owe in deductibles and copayments.

You have the right to call the hospital billing department and request a more detailed bill. To help decipher your bills, you have the right to obtain a copy of your medical records, including physician and nurses' notes, procedures, treatments, medications, and other tests.

6. Address billing concerns immediately.

If you have questions or concerns about the accuracy of your bill, immediately contact the provider's billing department. If you are not satisfied with the explanation, contact your insurance company, Medicare, or Medicaid as appropriate.

7. Appeal insurance denials.

An appeal is the action you can take if you disagree with a coverage or payment decision made by your insurance plan. The steps you must take depend on the type of insurance you have. If you have Medicare, a Medicare health plan, or Medicare Prescription Drug Plan, you may appeal any of the following denials:

- ✓ Request for a healthcare service, supply, item, or prescription drug to which you feel entitled;
- ✓ Request for payment of a healthcare service, supply, item, or prescription drug you previously received;
- ✓ Request to change the amount you must pay for a healthcare service, supply, item, or prescription drug.

You may also appeal if Medicare or your plan stops providing or paying for all or part of a healthcare service, supply, item, or prescription drug you think you still need.

You can find detailed information about the Medicare appeal process online at http://www.medicare.gov/claims-and-appeals/file-an-appeal/appeals.html or in the 2014 Medicare and You, available online at: http://www.medicare.gov/Pubs/pdf/10050.pdf or by calling Medicare at 1-800-Medicare.

The Affordable Care Act requires insurance companies to provide those it insures the right to a rigorous appeal process conducted by an independent entity.

8. Keep excellent records.

Keep copies of your billing statements and medical records. Document when and with whom you spoke about what issue. Having this information will be especially helpful if you file a complaint or an appeal.

Chapter 4
Discharge Rights

Medicaid and Medicare certified healthcare providers must follow federal regulations governing patient discharge procedures. These regulations require providers to:

➢ Comprehensively plan for the patient's safe discharge;

➢ Include the patient in the discharge planning process; and

➢ Where applicable, inform the patient of his right to appeal the discharge.

Hospital Patient Discharge Rights

To ensure the health and safety of patients, CMS requires hospitals to identify, at an early stage of hospitalization, patients who require discharge planning in order to avoid adverse health consequences. Patients who need the services of a home health agency (HHA) or skilled nursing care facility (SNF) after discharge, have the right to receive a list of Medicare certified HHAs and SNFs located near the patient.

If a patient is enrolled in a managed care organization (MCO), the hospital must advise of HHAs and SNFs that contract with the patient's MCO.

CMS prohibits hospitals from steering patients to certain HHA or SNFs. The patient (or the patient's family) has the right to choose among participating Medicare providers of post-hospital care services. The hospital must, to the extent possible, respect patient and family preferences when they are expressed. As discussed in Part I, the hospital must inform the patient if the hospital has a financial interest, such as ownership, in the HHA or SNF which appears on the list provided to the patient.[88]

Appealing a Medicare Beneficiary's Hospital Discharge

As discussed in Part I of this book, CMS has taken several steps to address the issue of hospital readmissions. One of those steps includes granting Medicare patients the right to appeal their discharge if they do not feel medically ready to leave the hospital.

CMS requires hospitals to inform Medicare beneficiaries of their right to appeal their hospital discharge by providing them with the Important Message from Medicare (IM).

Medicare beneficiaries have a right to request a review of their discharge by their state's Quality Improvement Organization (QIO). See Appendix D for a list of QIOs by state.

For those beneficiaries who request a QIO review, the hospital must deliver a Detailed Notice of Discharge as soon as possible, but no later than noon of the day after the QIO's notification. If a hospital fails to provide the beneficiary with the required notice, the hospital (not the beneficiary) may be held financially responsible for the patient's hospital stay.[89]

Ambulatory Surgical Center Patient Discharge Rights

CMS requires all Medicare certified Ambulatory Surgical Centers (ASCs) to ensure that patients are ready and prepared for discharge from the ASC. ASCs must provide patients with written discharge instructions and overnight supplies. When appropriate, ASCs must make patients' follow up appointments with the physician, and ensure that all patients are informed, either in advance of their surgical procedure or prior to leaving the ASC, of their prescriptions, post-operative instructions and physician contact information for follow-up care.

ASCs must ensure that patients have a discharge order, signed by the physician who performed the surgery or procedure. Additionally, ASCs must ensure all patients are discharged in the company of a responsible adult, except those patients exempted by the attending physician.[90]

Nursing Home Resident Discharge Rights

Federal regulations protect residents of nursing facilities from being inappropriately discharged by limiting the reasons for discharge, requiring nursing facilities to give residents 30-days' notice of discharge, and ensuring residents' right to appeal a discharge to the State Agency.

CMS prohibits facilities from discharging residents *except* for the following reasons:

- ➢ The transfer or discharge is necessary for the resident's welfare and the resident's needs cannot be met in the facility.
- ➢ The transfer or discharge is appropriate because the resident's health has improved sufficiently so the resident no longer needs the services provided by the facility.
- ➢ The safety of individuals in the facility is endangered.
- ➢ The health of individuals in the facility would otherwise be endangered.
- ➢ The resident has failed, after reasonable and appropriate notice, to pay for (or to have paid under Medicare or Medicaid) a stay at the facility.
- ➢ The facility ceases to operate.

In most cases, the resident has the right to be notified 30 days in advance of being transferred or discharged from the facility.

The discharge notice must include:

- ➢ the reason for transfer or discharge;
- ➢ the effective date of transfer or discharge;
- ➢ the location to which the resident is to be transferred or discharged;
- ➢ a statement that the resident has the right to appeal the action to the State;
- ➢ the name, address and telephone number of the State Long Term Care Ombudsman;
- ➢ (for nursing facility residents with developmental disabilities) the mailing address and telephone number of the agency responsible for the protection and advocacy of developmentally disabled individuals; and
- ➢ (for nursing facility residents who are mentally ill) the mailing address and telephone number of the agency responsible for the protection and advocacy of mentally ill individuals.[91]

State law governing nursing home care may provide additional protection against inappropriate transfer and discharge.

The resident has the right to appeal the discharge to the State's Survey Agency. Patients and their advocates may wish to contact their local Long Term Care Ombudsman or legal service agency for assistance with the appeal process.

Protecting Residents' Discharge Rights: The Case of the
"Disruptive" Nursing Home Resident.

Years ago in my role as consumer advocate, Ms. Jindell called me from the pay phone in the lobby of the nursing home where she lived. She found my number on the Long Term Care Ombudsman poster hanging on the bulletin board in the nursing home's activity room. She explained that the nursing home administrator told her that she was being discharged from the nursing home that day because of her disruptive behavior.   During the previous weeks, Ms. Jindell had parked herself by the home's entrance to advise anyone who entered what a "rat hole" the place was. She told visitors that the food was not fit for human consumption, the nursing assistants were incompetent, and the administrator was a "thief." Despite her disdain for the nursing home, she objected to the pending discharge, stating that she, not the administrator, would decide when it was time for her to leave. She wanted to know her rights and how to protect them.

I advised Ms. Jindell that the nursing home in which she lived was Medicare certified and licensed by the state. Therefore, the home was obligated to follow Medicare Conditions of Participation (CoPs) and state rules.

Specifically, the nursing home was required to provide Ms. Jindell a 30-day written notice of discharge detailing the reason for discharge, and Ms. Jindell's right to appeal.[92] Voicing one's opinion is not a legal reason for discharge. Once aware of her rights, Ms. Jindell was empowered to stave off the impermissible discharge, eventually transferring to another home of her choice in accordance with her desired time frame.

End Stage Renal Disease Facility Patient Discharge Rights

CMS requires End Stage Renal Disease (ESRD) facilities to inform patients of the facilities' policies for transfer, routine or involuntary discharge, and discontinuation of services to patients. Facilities must prominently display a copy of the patient's rights, including the current State Survey Agency and ESRD Network mailing addresses and telephone complaint numbers.

Patients have the right to receive a written notice 30 days in advance of an involuntary discharge, after the facility follows the involuntary discharge procedures described in 42 CFR §494.180(f)(4). In the case of immediate threats to the health and safety of others, an abbreviated discharge procedure may be allowed.

The ESRD Conditions for Coverage (CfCs) prohibit ESRD facilities from discharging patients *except* for the following reasons:

> ➤ The patient or payor no longer reimburses the facility for the ordered services;
> ➤ The facility ceases to operate;
> ➤ The transfer is necessary for the patient's welfare because the facility can no longer meet the patient's documented medical needs; or
> ➤ The facility has reassessed the patient and determined that the patient's behavior is disruptive and abusive to the extent that the delivery of care to the patient, or the ability of the facility to operate effectively, is seriously impaired. In this case, the patient's interdisciplinary team must:
>   - o Document the reassessments, ongoing problem(s), and efforts made to resolve the problem(s), and enter this documentation into the patient's medical record;
>   - o Provide the patient and the local ESRD Network with a 30-day notice of the planned discharge;
>   - o Obtain a written physician's order that must be signed by both the medical director and the patient's attending physician concurring with the patient's discharge or transfer from the facility;
>   - o Contact another facility, attempt to place the patient there, and document that effort; and
>   - o Notify the State Survey Agency of the involuntary transfer or discharge.[93]

Chapter 5

Right to Emergency Medical Treatment

In 1986, Congress enacted the Emergency Medical Treatment and Labor Act (EMTALA)[94] in response to incidents of "patient dumping." Because of a lack of medical insurance, patients were being denied emergency care, which sometimes resulted in patient death. Under EMTALA, a patient who comes to an emergency department seeking treatment has the right to a medical screening examination (MSE) and stabilizing treatment. The emergency department may not delay or deny the MSE or stabilizing treatment for discriminatory reasons such as the patient's inability to pay, race, gender, religion or sexual orientation.

Patients and their advocates have the right to file a formal grievance with the hospital if they were denied appropriate emergency care. CMS and the State Agency have authority to investigate EMTALA issues.

Chapter 6

Rights Related to
Durable Medical Equipment,
Prosthetics, Orthotics, and Supplies
(DMEPOS)

DMEPOS Quality Standards

Years ago in my role as consumer advocated I receive a phone call from Ms. Smith, a sixty year old woman who lived alone in the community. The automatic wheelchair she had been anticipating for over six months had finally arrived. When her last wheelchair stopped working, she lost her mobility and independence. She stopped volunteering at the community center, going out to eat with her friends, or wheeling to the end of her driveway to pick up her mail. The arrival of her new chair represented a return to freedom. Now she wept as she explained that "some guy in a white van" left the chair on her front porch and, even with the help of her neighbor, she could not get it to work. She said even if the chair had worked, it would not fit through her front door. There were no instructions with the chair. She called the phone number on the wheelchair invoice, but no one answered and there was no answering machine to leave a message.

Her only recourse, legal action against the company that provided the chair, soon became pointless since the company had closed its doors, leaving no forwarding address. She had to start again, paying out-of-pocket for a new wheelchair.

Had I received Ms. Smith's call today, we could have resolved the issue without relying on the legal system. In September 2010, CMS implemented regulations to protect Medicare consumers from such unscrupulous practices. Now, Medicare certified DMEPOS providers must comply with consumer protection requirements in order to be paid by Medicare.[95] These requirements affect the following types of DMEPOS suppliers:

- durable medical equipment (such as oxygen equipment and power wheelchairs);
- medical supplies (such as diabetic supplies);
- home dialysis supplies and equipment;
- therapeutic shoes;
- parenteral/enteral nutrition;
- transfusion medicine;
- prosthetic devices; and
- prosthetics and orthotics.

The requirements protect Medicare beneficiaries from shoddy products and service by requiring DMEPOS providers to be accredited and have a surety bond. In addition, DMEPOS providers must:

➢ Ensure that technical personnel are competent to deliver and set-up equipment, items and services, and train beneficiaries and/or caregivers;

➢ Provide information regarding expected time frames for receipt of items;

➢ Provide clear, written or pictorial, and verbal instructions related to the use, maintenance, infection control practices for, and potential hazards of equipment and items as appropriate;

➢ Verify that equipment, items and services were received;

➢ Document in the beneficiary's record the make and model number or any other identifier of any non-custom equipment and/or item(s) provided;

➢ Provide essential contact information for rental equipment and options for beneficiaries and/or caregivers to rent or purchase equipment;

➢ Provide information and telephone numbers for customer service, regular business hours, after-hours access, equipment and items repair, and emergency coverage; and

➢ Advise the ordering physician or other healthcare team member within five calendar days if the DME supplier cannot or will not provide the equipment, items or services.

Within five calendar days of receiving a beneficiary's complaint, the supplier must notify the beneficiary that it has received the complaint and is investigating. Within 14 calendar days of receiving a beneficiary's complaint, the supplier must provide written notification to the beneficiary of the results of its investigation.

Medicare Beneficiary Complaints about a DMEPOS Providers

DMEPOS suppliers must provide regular business hours and after-hour access telephone number(s) for customer service, and for information about equipment repair and emergency coverage. Beneficiaries and their advocates should attempt to resolve complaints directly with suppliers. However, if the issue is not resolved by the supplier, beneficiaries and their advocates may contact: Medicare at 1-800-MEDICARE (1-800-633-4227); or the State Health Insurance Assistance Program, or SHIP, which offers free local one-on-one counseling and assistance via telephone, or face-to-face for people with Medicare.[96]

Chapter 7

Right to Know about Medical Errors

Although healthcare providers are required to give quality care, the unfortunate truth is that providers make mistakes that harm patients. Healthcare providers are not mandated by federal regulation to tell patients about medical errors related to their care.

In 2001, The Joint Commission (then known as the Joint Commission on Accreditation of Healthcare Organizations) issued the first disclosure standard, requiring organizations to disclose unanticipated outcomes related to *sentinel events*. The Joint Commission defines a *sentinel event* as "an unexpected occurrence involving death or serious physical or psychological injury, or the risk thereof."[97]

In response, a majority of hospitals have some type of disclosure policy, but there is much debate as to the effectiveness of such policies.[98] Because providers fear litigation and/or harm to reputation, they are reluctant to advise patients and their families of medical errors.

As of 2010, thirty-four states and the District of Columbia have adopted "apology" laws, making apologies for medical mistakes inadmissible in court. Nine states have adopted "disclosure" laws to provide protection for those conversations.[99]

While the debate continues, patients and their families suffer when they do not receive a full explanation and appropriate compensation for harm caused by a medical error.[100] It is my belief that providers should be required by federal and state law to disclose adverse events to patients and their families. This data would assist all of us in our efforts to make informed decisions about our healthcare.

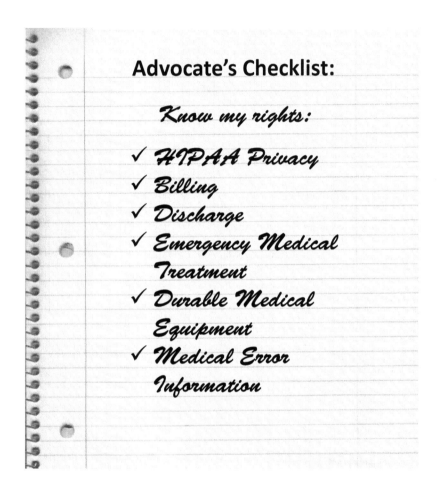

Advocate's Checklist:

Know my rights:

✓ *HIPAA Privacy*
✓ *Billing*
✓ *Discharge*
✓ *Emergency Medical Treatment*
✓ *Durable Medical Equipment*
✓ *Medical Error Information*

Part IV
Resolving Concerns

More than ever, healthcare providers want to promptly resolve the concerns of patients and their advocates.

First, providers know that dissatisfied patients not only take their business elsewhere, they shout their dissatisfaction from the mountain top of the Internet. In his fascinating book "Satisfied Customers Tell Three Friends, Angry Customers Tell 3,000," Pete Blackshaw chronicles the effect one disgruntled customer can have on a multi-billion dollar company. He cautions that unhappy patients can blog, network, or You Tube the best branding efforts down the drain.[101] In this day of increasing costs and decreasing reimbursement, healthcare providers cannot afford to let patients take their business elsewhere.

Second, dissatisfied patients answer satisfaction surveys negatively. As discussed in Part I of this book, CMS requires certain providers to survey patients about their healthcare experience. CMS then factors in those results when determining how much to pay providers. Low patient experience scores negatively affect providers' bottom line.

Third, healthcare providers are required by law to address patient concerns within a specific time frame and provide written follow-up. Failure to do so can result in regulatory citation and/or financial penalties.

The following discussion equips patients and their advocates to address issues in a timely and meaningful manner.   The most effective way to resolve patient concerns is to:

1. Know your rights
2. Speak calmly and confidently
3. Use the formal grievance process if needed
4. Participate in the resolution
5. Escalate the issue if necessary

1. Know Your Rights

The most powerful complaint resolution tool is a solid understanding of what the law requires of the healthcare provider. In this book, we have discussed the rules pertaining to some of the most common healthcare consumer concerns.   When a problem arises, take time to identify the issue and review what the provider is required by rule or regulation to do.   When providers realize that you know their obligations and your rights, they tune in to your concern.

Once you have a full understanding of what the healthcare provider is required to do, you must express that understanding in a calm and confident manner.

2. Speak Calmly and Confidently

It is easy to fly off the handle when you or someone you care about is not receiving appropriate care or treatment. Dealing with the complex, expensive, and sometimes impersonal world of healthcare can be emotionally overwhelming. This challenge, when coupled with exhaustion and worry over the patient's well-being, can create conflict.

Before you approach a healthcare provider with your concern, take time to calm down. If possible, take a walk, speak with a friend, or have a soothing drink.

It is not effective to start a conversation with the provider by threatening to sue. Most healthcare providers will stop the conversation and refer the matter to their legal counsel, essentially putting an end to the possibility of a timely or meaningful resolution. Yelling, swearing or threatening healthcare providers will likely quash communication and may result in a referral to the provider's Protective Services Officer. Here are some examples of effective and non-effective ways of stating the issue.

Ineffective	Effective
You people violated my HIPAA rights and I'll make sure you are closed down if it's the last thing I do.	HIPAA requires you to give me access to my records within 30 days of my request. We are at day 28 and I need you to help me resolve this so that I do not have to escalate the matter.
My mother sat in your emergency department waiting room for three hours and you treated everyone but her because she is on Medicaid.	Under EMTALA my mother has the right to a medical exam and stabilizing treatment without delay. She cannot be put at the end of the list because she does not have private insurance. I want a full investigation of the reason she waited three hours without being seen.

3. Use the Formal Grievance Process if Needed

Some concerns can be resolved quickly. For issues that require one or two steps to fix, it is best to go directly to the person who can resolve the problem. For instance, if the wrong meal tray is delivered to a hospital patient, a call to the dietary department or the charge nurse should be enough to get the correct tray. Likewise, if a nursing home resident needs clean sheets, advising a nursing assistant or supervisor may be all that is needed.

On the other hand, if the issue is persistent or complicated, you may need to file a formal grievance with the provider's manager or patient advocate.

CMS requires most Medicare certified providers to establish a formal grievance process to investigate and address patient complaints and grievances within a certain number of days. The process varies slightly depending on the type of provider. To know your grievance rights in all healthcare settings, see the regulations listed below. The Code of Federal Regulations (CFR) is accessible online at: http://www.ecfr.gov/cgi-bin/ECFR?page=browse

Patient Grievance Regulations by Provider Type	
Provider Type	*Regulation*
Ambulatory Surgical Center	42 CFR §416.50(1)(3)
End Stage Renal Disease	42 CFR §494.70(a)(14)-(17)
Home Health Care	42 CFR §484.10(b)
Hospice	42 CFR §418.25(b)
Hospital	42 CFR §482.13(b)
Long Term Care Facility	42 CFR §483.10(f)

The Hospital Grievance Process

Every Medicare certified hospital is required by law to establish a process for prompt resolution of patient grievances.[102]   A patient grievance is a written or verbal complaint by a patient or the patient's representative regarding:

> ➢ the patient's care;
> ➢ abuse or neglect;
> ➢ the hospital's compliance with the CMS Hospital Conditions of Participation (CoPs); or
> ➢ a Medicare beneficiary billing complaint related to rights and limitations provided by 42 CFR §489.

CMS so broadly defines grievance that most patient concerns fall into this category. For instance, "patient care" is a broad net that covers multiple patient concerns including, but not limited to, medication administration, inadequate hygiene, delay in call light response, or lack of medical information.

Examples of CoPs include: compliance with federal, state and local laws; patients' rights; discharge planning; quality assessment and performance; medical staff; nursing service; medical record service; pharmaceutical service; and radiological service.   The following chart describes what are and are not grievances.

Grievances	Non-Grievances
• Any patient care concern that cannot be resolved at the time of the concern by staff present, is postponed for later resolution, is referred to other staff for later resolution, requires investigation, and/or requires further actions for resolution • Any concern which a patient requests be handled as a formal complaint or grievance	• Concern resolved promptly by staff present
• Medicare billing/coverage issue	• Non-Medicare billing issue
• Patient survey response with an attached concern and request for resolution • Patient survey response with an attached concern which would normally be considered a grievance regardless of whether the patient requests resolution	• Patient survey response without an attached complaint and request for resolution
• Concern involving patient care • Concern alleging abuse or neglect • Concern pertaining to a hospital's compliance with CMS CoPs • Medicare beneficiary discharge dispute	

If the patient's issue meets the definition of grievance, CMS requires hospitals to investigate, resolve, and provide a written response for most grievances within an "appropriate time frame," defined generally as seven days.

If the grievance will not be resolved or the investigation will not be completed within seven days, CMS states that the hospital "should inform the patient or the patient's representative that the hospital will follow up with a written response within a stated number of days in accordance with the hospital's grievance policy." In any event, CMS states that a hospital should attempt to resolve all grievances as soon as possible.

CMS requires written follow-up for every grievance. In its resolution of the grievance, the hospital must provide the patient with written notice of its decision that contains:

> the name of the hospital contact person;
> the steps taken on behalf of the patient to investigate the grievance;
> the results of the grievance process; and
> the date of completion.[103]

4. Participate in the Resolution

For the best possible resolution, know and clearly describe your desired outcome. As Zig Ziglar is noted as saying: "If you aim at nothing, you will hit it every time." The desired outcome must be reasonable. Striving to "have the place shut down" or "get the entire staff fired" is not reasonable. It is reasonable to say, "I want my husband to receive the physical therapy the physician ordered during his hospital stay" or "I want your company's representative to fix or replace the broken wheel chair your company delivered yesterday."

Identify mutually agreeable resolution steps and a time frame for completing them. Take detailed notes describing when and with whom you spoke, the agreed upon next steps, and resolution time frame. Keep track of the progress and hold providers accountable for doing what they say they will do.

5. Escalate the Issue if Necessary

Most problems can be resolved directly with the healthcare provider by speaking with the manager responsible for the department or unit at issue. If the manager is not responsive and the formal grievance process does not resolve the issue, consider filing the complaint with one or more of the following organizations.

The Joint Commission. The Joint Commission, a national accrediting organization, will investigate quality of care complaints made against organizations it accredits. Complaints must be filed in writing. To learn more about filing a complaint with The Joint Commission, see: http://jcwebnoc.jcaho.org/QMSInternet/IncidentEntry.aspx.

Medicare Ombudsman. CMS established the Medicare Ombudsman to investigate and resolve complaints on behalf of beneficiaries. The Medicare Beneficiary Ombudsman Center is located online at: http://www.medicare.gov/navigation/help-and-support/ombudsman.aspx.

Quality Improvement Organization (QIO). QIOs work under the direction of CMS to investigate concerns on behalf of Medicare beneficiaries. Examples of quality of care concerns that the QIO can address are:

- ➢ medication errors;
- ➢ unnecessary or inappropriate surgery;
- ➢ unnecessary or inappropriate treatment;
- ➢ change in condition not treated;
- ➢ discharge from the hospital too soon; and
- ➢ incomplete discharge instructions and/or arrangements.

For more information about QIOs see: CMS Quality Net online at: http://www.qualitynet.org. See Appendix D of this book for a list of state QIOs.

Office for Civil Rights (OCR). The OCR of the U.S. Department of Health & Human Services (HHS) protects individuals from discrimination in certain healthcare and social service programs, such as hospitals, health clinics, and nursing homes. Individuals can file a discrimination complaint online at: http://www.hhs.gov/ocr/civilrights/complaints/index.html.

The OCR also enforces the HIPAA Privacy and Security Rules to protect individuals' health information held by health insurers and certain healthcare providers. Patients and their advocates may file HIPAA privacy complaints online with the OCR at: http://www.hhs.gov/ocr/privacy/hipaa/complaints/index.html.

Office of Inspector General (OIG). The OIG of the U.S. Department of Health & Human Services (HHS) conducts criminal, civil and administrative investigations of fraud and misconduct related to Medicare and Medicaid programs, operations and beneficiaries. The OIG Hotline accepts tips from all sources about potential fraud, waste, abuse, and mismanagement involving HHS programs. Consumers may contact the OIG online at: http://oig.hhs.gov/fraud/report-fraud/index.asp.

State Agency. CMS contracts with State Agencies to conduct annual surveys and complaint investigations involving certified healthcare organizations. A list of State Agencies and phone numbers can be found online at: http://www.hospitalcomplaint.com/stateagencies.html.

State Departments of Insurance. Each state's Department of Insurance is responsible for regulating and investigating complaints against insurance companies and their agents. A listing of state Departments of Insurance is available at the National Association of Insurance Commissioners website: http://www.naic.org/state_web_map.htm.

State Medical Board. The state medical board is responsible for licensing and regulating physicians and certain other healthcare professionals. Patients and advocates who have concerns about a doctor, such as unprofessional conduct, incompetent practice, or licensing, may contact their state medical board. A list of state medical boards can be found at the Federation of State Medical Boards website: http://www.fsmb.org/directory_smb.html.

Resolving Patient Care Complaints – Doctors Orders Not Followed

My 85-year-old mother was hospitalized following surgery. Her surgeon told her that he ordered daily physical therapy and it was essential that she participate in order to return home. He explained that she needed to get moving to avoid a blood clot and/or pneumonia and to strengthen her gait to prevent falling. Although my mother was ready and willing, the physical therapist failed to show for the next two days. When my mother asked the nurse about it, she replied that the physical therapists were busy and only had so many hours in their day. By noon on day three, the physical therapist still had not arrived and the nurse offered the same explanation – too much work, too little time.

My mother was discouraged and frustrated. With her permission, I contacted the hospital Ombudsman, whose job it is to help patients resolve issues. I described the issue and the Ombudsman explained there was nothing she could do and the physical therapists would arrive when their schedule allowed.

I told the Ombudsman, "Please relay this message to your senior leadership. The surgeon ordered daily physical therapy and three days have passed without it. Failure to provide physical therapy as ordered by the physician violates Medicare regulations. Knowingly accepting Medicare payment for care not provided is fraud. I intend to contact CMS."

Within the hour physical therapy arrived, providing therapy then and each day thereafter. Even the nurses offered to help my mom walk the hall. She was discharged within one week.

Advocate's Checklist:

To resolve concerns:

- ✓ *Know my rights*
- ✓ *Speak calmly and confidently*
- ✓ *Use the formal grievance process if needed*
- ✓ *Participate in the resolution*
- ✓ *Escalate the issue if necessary*

Conclusion

While one informed healthcare consumer improves his or her experience, a group of empowered advocates can help mend the healthcare system. In the words of Margaret Mead: "Never doubt that a small group of thoughtful, committed citizens can change the world. Indeed, it is the only thing that ever has."

Let each of us heed the call to become empowered advocates for ourselves and others. Let us pledge to actively participate in our healthcare, using available information to choose our providers, insurance plan, and alternate decision-makers. We must insist on price transparency so that we can make informed healthcare purchases and verify the accuracy of our medical bills. When we demand reliable information upon which to base our decisions, we spark market forces and increase provider accountability. We must commit to knowing our rights and holding providers accountable should they violate them.

When we demonstrate confidence in our knowledge and ability to navigate our healthcare journey, we have taken the first critical step toward healing.

Appendix A

Hospital Patient Rights CoP **42 CFR §482.13(a) – (h)**
A hospital must protect and promote each patient's rights.
A hospital must inform each patient, or when appropriate, the patient's representative (as allowed under State law), of the patient's rights, in advance of furnishing or discontinuing patient care whenever possible. This includes a hospital's duty to provide "An Important Message from Medicare" (IM), 42 CFR §489.27(b), (which cross references the regulation at 42 CFR 405.§1205 "Notifying beneficiaries of hospital discharge appeal rights").
The patient (or representative) has the right to be informed of the hospital's internal grievance process, including whom to contact to file a grievance (complaint). As part of its notification of patient rights, the hospital must provide the patient or the patient's representative a phone number and address for lodging a grievance with the State agency. The hospital must inform the patient that he/she may lodge a grievance with the State agency directly, regardless of whether he/she has first used the hospital's grievance process.
The patient has the right to participate in the development and implementation of his or her plan of care.
The patient or his or her representative has the right to make informed decisions regarding his or her care.
The patient has the right to be informed of his or her health status.
The patient has the right to be involved in care planning and treatment.
The patient has the right to formulate advance directives and to have hospital staff and practitioners who provide care in the hospital comply with these directives.
The patient has the right to have a family member or representative of his or her choice and his or her own physician notified promptly of his or her admission to the hospital.
The patient has the right to personal privacy.
The patient has the right to receive care in a safe setting.
The patient has the right to be free from all forms of abuse or harassment.

Hospital Patient Rights (Cont.)
The patient has the right to the confidentiality of his or her clinical records.
The patient has the right to access information contained in his or her clinical records within a reasonable time frame. The hospital must not frustrate the legitimate efforts of individuals to gain access to their own medical records and must actively seek to meet these requests as quickly as its record keeping system permits.
The patient has the right to receive visitors whom he or she designates, including, but not limited to, a spouse, a domestic partner (including a same-sex domestic partner), another family member, or a friend, and his or her right to withdraw or deny such consent at any time. 42 CFR §482.13(h) is available at: http://edocket.access.gpo.gov/2010/pdf/2010-29194.pdf.

Appendix B

Ambulatory Surgical Center (ASC) Patient Rights CfC, 42 CFR §416.50
ASC must inform the patient or the patient's representative or surrogate of the patient's rights and must protect and promote the exercise of these rights, as set forth in this section. The ASC must also post the written notice of patient rights in a place or places within the ASC likely to be noticed by patients waiting for treatment or by the patient's representative or surrogate, if applicable.
ASC must, prior to the start of the surgical procedure, provide the patient, the patient's representative, or the patient's surrogate with verbal and written notice of the patient's rights in a language and manner that ensures the patient, the representative, or the surrogate understand all of the patient's rights as set forth in this section. The ASC's notice of rights must include the address and telephone number of the State agency to which patients may report complaints, as well as the Web site for the Office of the Medicare Beneficiary Ombudsman.
An ASC that has physician owners or investors must provide written notice to the patient, the patient's representative or surrogate, prior to the start of the surgical procedure, that the ASC has physician-owners or physicians with a financial interest in the ASC.
Provide the patient or, as appropriate, the patient's representative with written information concerning its policies on advance directives, including a description of applicable State health and safety laws and, if requested, official State advance directive forms.
Inform the patient or, as appropriate, the patient's representative of the patient's right to make informed decisions regarding the patient's care.
The patient has the right to formulate advance directives.
The patient has the right to file a grievance.
The patient has the right to exercise his/her rights without being subjected to discrimination or reprisal.
The patient has the right to voice grievances regarding treatment or care that is (or fails to be) furnished.
The patient has the right to be fully informed about a treatment or procedure and the expected outcome before it is performed.

ASC Patient Rights (cont.)
The patient has a right to have his/her rights exercised by a person appointed under State law to act on the patient's behalf.
The patient has a right to have his/her rights exercised by a legal representative appointed by the patient.
The patient has the right to personal privacy.
The patient has a right to receive care in a safe setting.
The patient has the right to be free from all forms of abuse or harassment.
The patient has the right to confidential treatment of clinical records.

Appendix C

End Stage Renal Disease (ESRD) Facility Patient Rights CfCs 42 CFR §494.90
The patient has the right to respect, dignity, and recognition of his or her individuality and personal needs, and sensitivity to his or her psychological needs and ability to cope with ESRD.
The patient has the right to receive all information in a way that he or she can understand.
The patient has the right to privacy and confidentiality in all aspects of treatment.
The patient has the right to privacy and confidentiality in personal medical records.
The patient has the right to be informed about and participate, if desired, in all aspects of his or her care, and be informed of the right to refuse treatment, to discontinue treatment, and to refuse to participate in experimental research.
The patient has the right to be informed about his or her right to execute advance directives, and the facility's policy regarding advance directives.
The patient has the right to be informed about all treatment modalities and settings, including but not limited to, transplantation, home dialysis modalities (home hemodialysis, intermittent peritoneal dialysis, continuous ambulatory peritoneal dialysis, continuous cycling peritoneal dialysis),and in-facility hemodialysis. The patient has the right to receive resource information for dialysis modalities not offered by the facility, including information about alternative scheduling options for patients.
The patient has the right to be informed of facility policies regarding patient care, including, but not limited to, isolation of patients.
The patient has the right to be informed of facility policies regarding the reuse of dialysis supplies, including hemodialyzers
The patient has the right to be informed by the physician, nurse practitioner, clinical nurse specialist, or physician's assistant treating the patient for ESRD of his or her own medical status as documented in the patient's medical record, unless the medical record contains a documented contraindication.

ESRD Patient Rights (cont.)
The patient has the right to be informed of services available in the facility and charges for services not covered under Medicare.
The patient has the right to receive the necessary services outlined in the patient plan of care.
The patient has the right to be informed of the rules and expectations of the facility regarding patient conduct and responsibilities.
The patient has the right to be informed of the facility's internal grievance process.
The patient has the right to be informed of external grievance mechanisms and processes, including how to contact the ESRD Network and the State survey agency.
The patient has the right to be informed of his or her right to file internal grievances or external grievances or both without reprisal or denial of services.

Appendix D
Quality Improvement Organizations
Source: CMS Quality Net: http://www.qualitynet.org

State	Organization and Website Link	Telephone Number
Alabama	AQAF www.aqaf.com	205-970-1600
Alaska	Mountain-Pacific Quality Health www.mpqhf.org	800-497-8232
Arizona	Health Services Advisory Group, Inc. www.hsag.com	602-264-6382
Arkansas	Arkansas Foundation for Medical Care www.afmc.org	501-375-5700
California	Health Services Advisory Group of California, Inc. www.hsag.com	818-265-4650
Colorado	Colorado Foundation for Medical Care www.cfmc.org	303-695-3300
Connecticut	Qualidigm www.qualidigm.org	860-632-2008
Delaware	Quality Insights of Delaware www.qide.org	302-478-3600
District of Columbia	Delmarva Foundation of the District of Columbia www.dcqio.org	202-293-9650
Florida	FMQAI www.fmqai.com	800-564-7490
Georgia	Georgia Medical Care Foundation (GMCF) www.gmcf.org	404-982-0411
Hawaii	Mountain-Pacific Quality Health www.mpqhf.org	800-497-8232
Idaho	Qualis Health www.qualishealthmedicare.org	800-488-1118
Illinois	Telligen Illinois www.telligenqio.org	800-386-6431
Indiana	Health Care Excel www.hce.org	812-234-1499
Iowa	Telligen www.telligenqio.org	800-383-2856
Kansas	Kansas Foundation for Medical Care, Inc. www.kfmc.org	800-432-0407
Kentucky	Health Care Excel www.hce.org	502-454-5112
Louisiana	eQHealth Solutions louisianaqio.eqhs.org	225-926-6353

QIO (cont.)		
Maine	Northeast Health Care Quality Foundation www.nhcqf.org	800-772-0151
Maryland	Delmarva Foundation for Medical Care www.mdqio.org	443-285-0190
Massachusetts	Masspro www.masspro.org	781-890-0011
Michigan	MPRO www.mpro.org	248-465-7300
Minnesota	Stratis Health www.stratishealth.org	877-787-2847
Mississippi	Information & Quality Healthcare www.msqio.org	601-957-1575
Missouri	Primaris www.primaris.org	800-735-6776
Montana	Mountain-Pacific Quality Health www.mpqhf.org	800-497-8232
Nebraska	CIMRO of Nebraska www.cimronebraska.org	800-458-4262
Nevada	HealthInsight www.healthinsight.org	702-385-9933
New Hampshire	Northeast Health Care Quality Foundation www.nhcqf.org	800-772-0151
New Jersey	Healthcare Quality Strategies, Inc. www.hqsi.org	732-238-5570
New Mexico	New Mexico Medical Review Association www.nmmra.org	800-663-6351
New York	IPRO www.ipro.org	516-326-7767
North Carolina	The Carolinas Center for Medical Excellence www.ccmemedicare.org	800-682-2650
North Dakota	North Dakota Health Care Review, Inc. www.ndhcri.org	701-852-4231
Ohio	Ohio KePRO www.ohiokepro.com	800-385-5080
Oklahoma	Oklahoma Foundation for Medical Quality www.ofmq.com	405-840-2891
Oregon	Acumentra Health www.acumentra.org	503-279-0100
Pennsylvania	Quality Insights of Pennsylvania www.qipa.org	877-346-6180

QIO (cont.)		
Puerto Rico	Quality Improvement Professional Research Organization, Inc. www.qipro.org	787-641-1240
Rhode Island	Healthcentric Advisors www.healthcentricadvisors.org	401-528-3200
South Carolina	The Carolinas Center for Medical Excellence www.ccmemedicare.org	800-922-3089
South Dakota	South Dakota Foundation for Medical Care www.sdfmc.org	605-336-3505
Tennessee	QSource www.qsource.org	800-528-2655
Texas	TMF Health Quality Institute www.tmf.org	800-725-9216
Utah	HealthInsight www.healthinsight.org	801-892-0155
Vermont	Northeast Health Care Quality Foundation www.nhcqf.org	800-772-0151
Virgin Islands	Virgin Islands Medical Institute, Inc. www.viqio.org	340-712-2400
Virginia	VHQC www.vhqc.org	804-289-5320
Washington	Qualis Health www.qualishealthmedicare.org	800-949-7536
West Virginia	WVMI Quality Insights www.qiwv.org	800-642-8686
Wisconsin	MetaStar, Inc. www.metastar.com	800-362-2320
Wyoming	Mountain-Pacific Quality Health www.mpqhf.org	877-810-6248

Notes

---

[1] James, Julia. (Oct. 11, 2012). Pay-for-Performance. *Health Affairs*, 33: 8. Retrieved from http://www.healthaffairs.org/healthpolicybriefs/brief.php?brief_id=78

[2] Institute of Medicine. *To err is human: Building a safer health system.* Washington D.C.: National Academies Press, 2000

[3] Patient Protection and Affordable Care Act, 42 U.S.C. § 18001 et seq. (2010). Retrieved from http://www.gpo.gov/fdsys/pkg/PLAW-111publ148/content-detail.html

[4] The clinical outcome measures that eligible hospitals must report in 2014 are detailed online at: http://www.cms.gov/Regulations-and-Guidance/Legislation/EHRIncentivePrograms/Downloads/eCQM_EH_Table_April2014.pdf

[5] For more information about the HCAHPS survey process, see: http://www.hcahpsonline.org/files/August%202013%20HCAHPS%20Fact%20Sheet2.pdf

[6] The HCAHPS tool can be found at: http://www.hcahpsonline.org/files/HCAHPS%20V9.0%20Appendix%20A%20-%20Mail%20Survey%20Materials%20(English)%20March%202014.pdf

[7] The CAHPS Clinician and Group surveys are available at: https://www.cahps.ahrq.gov/surveys-guidance/survey2.0-docs/1351a_Adult12mo_Eng_20.pdf

[8] National Quality Forum (NQF), *Serious Reportable Events in Healthcare: A Consensus Report,* Washington, DC: NQF; 2002

[9] CMS. Inpatient Prospective Payment System (IPPS) Fiscal Year (FY) 2013 Final Rule

[10]Medicare Payment Advisory Commission: Payment Policy for Inpatient Readmissions: *Promoting Greater Efficiency in Medicare*. Report to Congress. June 2007.

[11]http://www.medicare.gov/hospitalcompare/Data/30-day-measures.html

[12] Information about the CMS readmission reduction program is available at: http://www.cms.gov/Medicare/Medicare-Fee-for-Service-Payment/AcuteInpatientPPS/Readmissions-Reduction-Program.html

[13]The Medicare Payment Advisory Commission. (June 2013) *Report to Congress: Medicare and the Health Care Delivery System*. Retrieved from http://medpac.gov/documents/reports/jun13_ch04.pdf?sfvrsn=0

[14] Information taken directly from the CMS Hospital Compare website page http://www.medicare.gov/hospitalcompare/About/Hospital-Info.html

[15] The Home Health Quality Measures are based on data from the Outcome and Assessment Information Set (OASIS) quality data submitted by home health agencies to state repositories and stored in the Quality Improvement Evaluation System (QIES) database. For more information see: https://homehealthcahps.org/Default.aspx?tabid=88

[16]The information on Dialysis Facility Compare comes from the National Claims History Standard Analytical Files (NCH SAFs) and Consolidated Renal Operations in a Web-enabled Network (CROWN). For more information see: http://www.medicare.gov/DialysisFacilityCompare/Data/Data-Sources.html

[17]The lack of price transparency is chronicled by Steven Brill in his article "Bitter Pill: Why Medical Bills are Killing Us." *Time*. 4 Mar 2013: 16-55.

[18] The Kaiser Family Foundation and Health Research & Educational Trust, *Employee Health Benefits 2013 Annual Survey* (2013). Retrieved from http://kaiserfamilyfoundation.files.wordpress.com/2013/08/8465-employer-health-benefits-20131.pdf

[19] *Health Care Transparency: Meaningful Price Information is Difficult for Consumers to Obtain Prior to Receiving Care.* (GAO Publication No. 11-791). Washington, D.C.: U.S. Government Printing Office

[20] PPACA, § 1001, 124 Stat. 119, 130-8, amended by §10101(f), 124 Stat. 119, 885-7 (codified in 42 U.S.C. § 300gg-18)

[21] Medicare payment data is available on line at: http://archive.hhs.gov/valuedriven/fourcornerstones/price/index.htm

[22] The Catalyst for Payment Reform. (March 2014). *Report Card on State Price Transparency Laws.* Retrieved from http://www.hci3.org/sites/default/files/files/Report_PriceTransLaws_2014.pdf

[23] Institute of Medicine (US) Committee on Conflict of Interest in Medical Research, Education, and Practice; Lo B, Field MJ, editors. Conflict of Interest in Medical Research, Education, and Practice. Washington (DC): National Academies Press (US); 2009. 6, Conflicts of Interest and Medical Practice. Available from: http://www.ncbi.nlm.nih.gov/books/NBK22944/

[24] For more information regarding the posting of physician payments, see the CMS website: http://www.cms.gov/Regulations-and-Guidance/Legislation/National-Physician-Payment-Transparency-Program/Public-Access-to-Data.html

[25] *Additional Requirements Concerning Physician Ownership and Investment in Hospitals* is codified in 42 CFR §411.362. See also: http://www.cms.gov/outreach-and-education/medicare-learning-network-mln/mlnmattersarticles/downloads/SE1332.pdf

[26] The Hospital Discharge Condition of Participation (CoP) is codified in 42 CFR §482. 43

[27]Consumer Reports. (March 2014). How to Pick a Health Insurance Plan: Three Most Important Questions You Need to Ask. Retrieved from http://www.consumerreports.org/cro/2012/09/understanding-health-insurance/index.htm

[28]Habilitative means "Health care services that help you keep, learn, or improve skills and functioning for daily living. Examples include therapy for a child who isn't walking or talking at the expected age. These services may include physical and occupational therapy, speech-language pathology, and other services for people with disabilities in a variety of inpatient and/or outpatient settings." Source: Healthcare.gov

[29] Patient Protection and Affordable Care Act, 42 U.S.C. §1302 (2010)

[30] For detailed pricing and comparison of the Affordable Care Act metal plans, see http://www.healthpocket.com/healthcare-research/infostat/2014-obamacare-deductible-out-of-pocket-costs/#.UyidUlzLtCN

[31] CMS Hospital CoPs address informed consent in several sections including: patient rights [42 CFR §482.13(b)(2)]; surgical services [42 CFR §482.51(b)(2)] and medical records [42 CFR §482.24(c)(4)]. CMS requires providers to maintain written documentation as evidence that informed consent was obtained

[32]Provider requirements pertaining to advance directives are codified in 42 CFR §489.102

[33]Anand, Preetha, Kunnumakara, Ajaikumar, et al. (Sept. 2008) Cancer is a Preventable Disease that Requires Major Lifestyle Changes. *Pharmaceutical Research*. 25:9, 2097-2116 Retrieved from http://www.ncbi.nlm.nih.gov/pmc/articles/PMC2515569/

[34] Visit the American Cancer Society website "Staying Healthy" web page at: http://www.cancer.org/healthy/index

[35] Visit the Centers for Disease Control and Prevention "Healthy Living" page at: http://www.cdc.gov/family/healthyliving/index.htm

[36] Visit the Harvard School of Public Health "Nutrition" and "Disease Prevention" pages at: http://www.hsph.harvard.edu/nutritionsource/disease-prevention/

[37] Agency for Healthcare Research and Quality (AHRQ). (Sept. 15, 2005) *Guide to Health Care Quality: How to Know It When You See It.* Retrieved from http://www.hr.tcu.edu/HealthcareQuality.pdf

[38] A List of CMS-approved Accreditation Organizations can be obtained at: http://www.cms.gov/SurveyCertificationGenInfo/Downloads/AOContactInformation.pdf

[39] Long Term Facilities Quality of Care CoP is codified in 42 CFR §483.25.

[40] Annual Report to Congress on Breaches of Unsecured Protected Health Information for Calendar Years 2009 and 2010, available on line at: http://www.hhs.gov/ocr/privacy/hipaa/administrative/breachnotificationrule/breachrept.pdf

[41] Id. at page 6

[42] The National Health Care Anti-Fraud Association. (Oct. 6, 2010) *Combating Health Care Fraud in a Post-Reform World: Seven Guiding Principles for Policy Makers.* Retrieved from http://www.nhcaa.org/media/5994/whitepaper_oct10.pdf

[43] FBI. Financial Crimes Report to the Public. Fiscal Years 2010-2011 Retrieved from http://www.fbi.gov/stats-services/publications/financial-crimes-report-2010-2011

[44] The OCR HIPAA enforcement data is available on line at: http://www.hhs.gov/ocr/privacy/hipaa/enforcement/data/top5issues. html.

[45] These and other examples of the OCR enforcement actions are found online at: http://www.hhs.gov/ocr/privacy/hipaa/enforcement/examples/allcas es.html#case17.

[46] 45 CFR §160.103

[47] The official title of the "Final Rule" is "Modifications to the HIPAA Privacy, Security, Enforcement, and Breach Notification Rules under the Health Information Technology for Economic and Clinical Health Act and the Genetic Information Nondiscrimination Act; Other Modifications to the HIPAA Rules" (Omnibus Rule), 78 Fed. Reg. 5566 (Jan. 25, 2013).

[48] The combined text of the Privacy and Security Rule is available on line at: http://www.hhs.gov/ocr/privacy/hipaa/administrative/combined/hipa a-simplification-201303.pdf.

[49] 45 CFR §164.308(b)(2)

[50]See the OCR guidance on de-identifying information, available on line at: http://www.hhs.gov/ocr/privacy/hipaa/understanding/coveredentitie s/De-identification/guidance.html

[51] 45 CFR §164.508(a)(2)

[52] 45 CFR §164.508(a)(3)

[53] 45 CFR §164.508(a)(4)

[54] The HITECH Final Rule specifically includes genetic information in the definition of protected health information (PHI) and prohibits use or disclosure of genetic information for underwriting purposes. See 45 CRF §164.502(a)(5).

[55] 45 CFR §164.508(a)(2)

[56] 42 CFR Part 2.

[57] 45 CFR §164.520

[58] 45 CFR §164.520(b)

[59] 45 CFR §164.524

[60] 45 CFR §164.526

[61] 45 CFR §164.528

[62] 45 CFR §164.522

[63] 45 CFR §164.522(b)(1)

[64] 45 CFR §164.514(f)

[65] 45 CFR §164.510

[66] 45 CFR §164.508(a)(3)

[67] 45 CFR §164.404

[68] This and other information about medical identity theft is available at the Federal Trade Commission website: http://www.consumer.ftc.gov/articles/0171-medical-identity-theft#Detecting.

[69] FBI, Financial Crimes Report to the Public. Fiscal Years 2010-2011. Retrieved from http://www.fbi.gov/stats-services/publications/financial-crimes-report-2010-2011

[70] 164 CFR §530(d)

[71] 164 CFR §530(a)(1)(ii)

[72] 164 CFR §530(e)

[73] 164 CFR §530(g)

[74] The OCR Cignet Health Civil Monetary Penalty announcement is available on line at: http://www.hhs.gov/ocr/privacy/hipaa/enforcement/examples/cignet cmp.html.

[75] The Red Flags Rule is available on line at: https://www.federalregister.gov/articles/2013/04/19/2013-08830/identity-theft-red-flags-rules.

[76] Brill, Steven. "Bitter Pill: Why Medical Bills are Killing Us." *Time* March 4, 2013: 16-55

[77] Palmer, Pat. *Medical Billing Errors Can Make Your Life a Nightmare.* Retrieved from the Medical Billing Advocates of America website, http://billadvocates.com/resources/medical-billing-errors-can-make-life-nightmare/

[78] American Medical Association. *Efforts with Health Insurers Cut Medical Claims Errors by Half.* June 12, 2012. Retrieved from http://www.ama-assn.org/ama/pub/news/news/2012-06-18-national-health-insurer-report-card.page

[79] CMS. Medicare Composite Benchmark Metric Report March 31, 2011. Retrieved from http://www.cms.gov/Medicare/Medicare-Contracting/Medicare-Administrative-Contractors/RedactedBenchmarkMetricReports.html.

[80] For detailed explanation of ABN requirements, see
http://www.cms.gov/bni/

[81] Provider-based requirements are codified in 42 CFR §413.65

[82] A Medicare beneficiary's billing issue is a grievance if it involves rights and limitations provided by 42 CFR §498. By incorporating by reference 42 CFR §498, CMS essentially mandates that any Medicare beneficiary billing concern is a grievance. Among other things, 42 CFR §498 specifies basic commitments and limitations to which Medicare providers must comply as part of an agreement to provide services. This includes the limitations on allowable charges to beneficiaries for deductibles, coinsurance, copayments, and services.
See 42 CFR 482.13(a)(2) Interpretive Guidelines

[83] For a detailed explanation of Medicare's prohibition against balance billing see the Boccuti, Cristina. Kaiser Family Foundation. Apr. 7, 2014. *Paying a Visit to the Doctor: Current Financial Protections for Medicare Patients When Receiving Physician Services*. Retrieved from http://kff.org/medicare/issue-brief/paying-a-visit-to-the-doctor-current-financial-protections-for-medicare-patients-when-receiving-physician-services/

[84] Section 1902(n)(3)(B) of the Social Security Act, as modified by 4714 of the Balanced Budget Act of 1997, prohibits Medicare from balance billing Qualified Medicare Beneficiaries (QMB) for Medicare cost-sharing. QMBs are individuals entitled to Medicare Part A and/or Part B and are eligible Medicaid

[85] For information on state prohibition of balance billing and managed care organizations see the Kaiser Family Foundation. *State Restrictions Against Providers Balance Billing Managed Care Enrollees*. 2013. Retrieved from http://kff.org/private-insurance/state-indicator/state-restriction-against-providers-balance-billing-managed-care-enrollees/

[86] Consumer Reports. *Check Medical Bills for Errors*. August, 2009. Retrieved from http://www.consumerreports.org/cro/money/personal-investing/check-medical-bills-for-errors/overview/index.htm

[87] Palmer, Pat. *10 Medical Billing Overcharges to Blow the Whistle On*. Retrieved from the Medical Billing Advocates of America website, http://billadvocates.com/resources/10-medical-billing-overcharges/

[88] Hospital Discharge CoP is codified in 42 CFR § 482.43

[89] Additional information on the CMS Hospital Discharge Appeal Notice is available at: http://www.cms.gov/Medicare/Medicare-General-Information/BNI/HospitalDischargeAppealNotices.html

[90] The ASC Patient Admission, Assessment and Discharge Condition for Coverage (CfC) is codified in 42 CFR §416.52

[91] Long Term Care Facility Admission, Transfer and Discharge Rights CoP is codified in 42 CFR § 483.12

[92] The Long Term Care CoP pertaining to discharge rights is codified in 42 CFR §483.12

[93] The ESRD Patient Rights CoP is codified in 42 CFR §494.70; The Involuntary Discharge and Transfer Policies and Procedures standard is codified in 42 CFR §494.180(f).

[94] 42 U.S.C. §1395dd . EMTALA can be found online at: http://www.cms.gov/Regulations-and-Guidance/Legislation/EMTALA/

[95] DMEPOS Quality Standards are available online at: http://www.cms.gov/MLNProducts/downloads/DMEPOS_Qual_Stand_Booklet_ICN905709.pdf.

[96] Additional information about SHIP, including state by state SHIP contacts, is available online at: http://www.cms.gov/Partnerships/10SHIPS.asp

[97]The Joint Commission. Sentinel Event Policy. Comprehensive Accreditation Manual for Hospitals March, 2013

[98] Barbara Phillips-Bute, Ph.D.,*Transparency and Disclosure of Medical Errors: It's the Right Thing to Do, So Why the Reluctance?*, 35 Campbell L. Rev. 333 (2014). Retrieved from http://scholarship.law.campbell.edu/clr/vol35/iss3/3/

[99]Anna C. Mastroianni et al., *The Flaws in State "Apology" and "Disclosure" Laws Dilute Their Intended Impact on Malpractice Suits,* Health Affairs, Sept. 2010 vol. 29 no. 9, 1611-1619. Retrieved from http://content.healthaffairs.org/content/29/9/1611.full

[100] For additional information regarding the disclosure debate, see the American Society for Healthcare Risk Management. *Disclosure of Unanticipated Events in 2013.* Retrieved from http://www.ashrm.org/ashrm/education/development/monographs/Disclosure-of-Unanticipated-Events-in-2013_Prologue.pdf

[101] Blackshaw, P. (2008). *Satisfied Customers Tell Three Friends, Angry Customers Tell 3,000.* New York, NY: Crown Business

[102]42 CFR §482.13(a)(2)

[103] 42 CFR §482.13(a)(2)(iii)

Made in the USA
Charleston, SC
11 April 2015